EYE ACUPUNCTURE THERAPY

Chief Editor　Zhao Xin
Translator　　Wang Tai

Academy Press [Xue Yuan]

First Edition 1997
ISBN 7 – 5077 – 1364 – 4

EYE ACUPUNCTURE THERAPY
Chief Editor   Zhao Xin
Translator   Wang Tai

Published by
Academy Press [Xue Yuan]
11 Wanshoulu Xijie, Beijing 100036, China

Distributed by
China International Book Trading Corporation
35 Chegongzhuang Xilu, Beijing, 100044, China
P.O. Box 399, Beijing China

Printed in the People's Republic of China

FOREWORD

In recent years, according to the theory of differential diagnosis of syndromes and the principle of selection of acupoints by inspection of blood vessels on eye, the eye acupuncture at acupoints around eyeball and on orbital edge to treat various general diseases of human beings has been used in clinical practice with a good therapeutic effect.

The eye acupuncture therapy was thoroughly discussed in 2 parts of this book. In the first part of the book, the basic theories of eye acupuncture were introduced and in the second part the definition, etiology, pathogenesis, differential diagnosis, treatment and clinical experience of more than 50 common diseases were mentioned as a reference for clinical practice of eye acupuncture therapy in traditional Chinese medicine.

From the author
Feb. 9, 1997

CONTENTS

PART 1 INTRODUCTION

I Theoretical Basis of Eye Acupuncture Therapy
.... (8)
1. Relation between eye and meridians ...... (8)
   (1) Relation between eye and 12 meridians ...
   .... (9)
   (2) Relation between eye and 8 extra meridians
   .... (13)
   (3) Relation between eye and meridianal muscles .... (16)
   (4) Relation between meridians and diseases
   .... (19)
2. Relation between eye and internal organs
   .... (23)
   (1) Relation between eye and heart and small intestine .... (23)
   (2) Relation between eye and liver and gallbladder .... (25)

  (3) Relation between eye and spleen and stomach ································· (26)
  (4) Relation between eye and lung and large intestine ································ (28)
  (5) Relation between eye and kidney and urinary bladder ······························ (29)
  (6) Relation between eye and triple energizer ·· (31)
  (7) Introduction of five wheel theory ··· (32)
 3. Anatomy of eye ···························· (38)

II Divisions of Eye ······························· (40)
 1. Divisions of 8 Diagrams ···················· (40)
 2. Mingmen (life gate) and Sanjiao (triple energizer) ······································· (43)
 3. Divisions of eye and relation with internal organs ······································· (49)
 4. Rememberance of eye diagram ············· (54)

III Location and Indications of Regions of Eye
································· (57)

IV Inspection of Eye for Diagnosis of Diseases
································· (62)

V Selection of Eye Acupoints .... (66)
  1. Selection of acupoints according to meridians
.... (66)
  2. Selection of acupoints according to abnormal change of blood vessels .... (66)
  3. Selection of acupoints in Sanjiao region ... (67)
  4. Localization of acupoints .... (68)

VI Practice of Acupuncture .... (68)

VII Methods of Eye Acupuncture .... (69)

VIII Needling Sensation and Techniques of Reinforcement and Reduction .... (73)

IX Retention and Removal of Needle ...... (74)
X Cautions .... (75)

PART 2 TREATMENT OF DISEASES

1. Common cold ·· (76)
2. Aphonia ··· (78)
3. Bronchial asthma ·· (80)
4. Cough ·· (83)
5. Vomiting ·· (86)
6. Hiccup ··· (89)
7. Stomachache ·· (92)
8. Jaundice ··· (95)
9. Cholelithiasis ·· (98)
10. Abdominal pain ·· (100)
11. Diarrhea ··· (102)
12. Constipation ··· (106)
13. Prolapse of rectum ·· (108)
14. Hypertensive disease ····································· (110)
15. Palpitation of heart ······································· (112)
16. Xiongbi (chest pain) ····································· (114)
17. Angina pectoris ··· (116)
18. Edema ·· (118)
19. Headache ·· (123)
20. Facial palsy ··· (128)
21. Apoplexy (stroke) ··· (130)

22. Insomnia ………………………………… (135)
23. Vertigo ……………………………………… (138)
24. Emission of semen ……………………… (141)
25. Impotence ………………………………… (144)
26. Stiff neck ………………………………… (145)
27. Trigeminal neuralgia …………………… (147)
28. Intercostal neuralgia …………………… (149)
29. Neuralgia sciatica ……………………… (150)
30. Lumbago …………………………………… (153)
31. Periarthritis of shoulder (frozen shoulder)
    …………………………………………………… (156)
32. Wei-syndrome (paralysis) ……………… (158)
33. Bi-syndrome (arthritis) ………………… (161)
34. Sprain of soft tissues …………………… (164)
35. Irregular menstruation ………………… (165)
36. Dysmenorrhea …………………………… (168)
37. Hyperemesis gravidarum ……………… (172)
38. Oligogalactia (reduction of milk secretion)
    …………………………………………………… (174)
39. Incontinence of urine (bed wetting)
    …………………………………………………… (176)
40. Urticaria …………………………………… (179)
41. Eczema ……………………………………… (181)
42. Furuncle and carbuncle ………………… (183)

43. Hemorrhoids ································ (185)
44. Ptosis of eyelid ···························· (187)
45. Strabismus (wall-eye) ······················ (189)
46. Hordeolum (stye) ·························· (191)
47. Red eye (conjunctivitis) ··················· (193)
48. Induction of lachrymation by wind
   ·· (195)
49. Qingmang (optic atrophy) ················· (196)
50. Tinnitus and deafness ····················· (198)
51. Biyuan (sinusitis) ·························· (202)
52. Sore throat ································· (204)
53. Toothache ·································· (207)
54. Febrile diseases ···························· (209)
55. Juesyndrome (syncope) ···················· (212)
56. Jingsyndrome (epilepsy) ··················· (215)
57. Tongsyndrome (painful diseases) ··········· (217)
58. Fig ··· (220)

PART 1   INTRODUCTION

The eye acupuncture therapy is used to treat diseases by applying acupuncure at the acupoints around the eyeball and on orbital edge and it is developed from the "diagnostic methods of diseases by inspecting eyes" established by Hua Tuo (a famous ancient physician in Han dynasty) and after analyzing and summarizing the clinical observation and treatment of physicians in following successive dynasties.

After a diagnosis is made by observing the minute changes of blood vessels on conjunctiva of eye, the acupoints around the eyes are selected according to the principle of differential diagnosis and treatment in traditional Chinese medicine to treat various diseases, such as acute muscular sprain, early stage of apoplexy (stroke) with hemiplegia and diseases of pain with a good therapeutic effect.

I Theoretical Basis of Eye Acupuncture Therapy

1. Relation between eye and meridians

The origins or terminals of 8 out of 12 meridians (except lung, spleen, kidney and pericardium meridians) are located in the region around the eye, but the latter 4 meridians have an indirect connection with the eye through a linkage with their exterointeriorly correlated meridians. As mentioned in Miraculous Pivot, a classical ancient medical book: "The essence of all internal organs can be supplied to eyes···"; "the blood and qi of 12 meridians and 365 collaterals can be supplied to the orifices on face; and the Yang qi is supplied to eyes to produce the essence of eyes"; and as mentioned in Plain Questions, another classical ancient medical book: "All meridians are connected with eyes." Therefore, the eyes are closely related to the internal organs and merididans and the acupuncture applied at the acupoints around eye can be used to treat many diseases of the whole body.

The meridians can connect all organs and structures of the body and supply qi and blood to them. As mentioned in Miraculous Pivot: "The eye is an organ to which all meridians assemble." Therefore, the eyes are closely connected with meridians and through them the qi and blood are supplied to eyes to keep a good vision.

(1) Relation between eye and 12 meridians

The 12 meridians are connected one by one in sequence from hand Taiyin to foot Jueyin meridian to form a closed circuit to transport Ying (nutrient) and blood. The Yang and Yin meridians are composed in pairs with an exterointeriorly correlated relationship with each other. Therefore, the eye is directly or indirectly connected with all 12 meridians.

The meridians passing through head and face and connected with eye are mentioned as follows:

1) Hand Yangming large intestine meridian: A branch of this meridian goes up to face and across to opposite side at Renzhong (GV 26) acupoint, passes around nostril and through Heliao (LI 19) acupoint and finally stops at Yingxiang (LI 20) acupoint below eye and beside nose to connect foot Yangming stomach meridian.

2) Foot Yangming stomach meridian: This meridian originates from Yingxiang (LI 20) acupoint beside

nose, goes up to Jingming (BL 1) acupoint after across nose bridge to connect foot Taiyang meridian and then it goes downward beside nose and through Chengqi (ST 1), Sibai (ST 2) and Juliao (ST 3) acupoints and finally enters the upper teeth. The main branch of this meridian also goes up through nose bridge and orbital edge to connect Muxi (tie of eye, including optic nerve and extra-ocular muscles).

3) Hand Shaoyin heart meridian: A branch of this meridian goes upward from Xinxi (tie of heart, including aorta and other big blood vessels) through throat to Muxi (tie of eye). A big collateral of this meridian, called Tongli also goes up to conncet Muxi (tie of eye). In addition, a main branch of this meridian goes up through face to connect a branch of hand Taiyang meridian at Jingming (BL 1) beside inner canthus of eye.

4) Hand Taiyang small intestine meridian: A branch of this meridian goes up through neck to Quanliao (SI 18) acupoint, passes through outer canthus of eye and Tongziliao (GB 1) acupoint and finally enters the ear. Another branch passes from cheek through lower border of orbit to Jingming (BL 1) acupoint beside inner canthus of eye to connect foot Taiyang merid-

ian.

5) Foot Taiyang urinary bladder meridian: The main branch of this meridian originates from Jingming (BL 1) beside inner canthus of eye and goes upward through Cuanzhu (BL 2), Shenting (GV 24) and Tongtian (BL 7) acupoints to connect Governor vessel at Baihui (GV 20) acupoint. A straight branch enters brain to connect Muxi (tie of eye).

6) Hand Shaoyang tripple energizer meridian: A branch of this meridian goes upward from chest through nape and Yifeng (TE 17) acupoint behind ear to Jiaosun (TE 20) acupoint at apex of ear and then goes downward through Yangbai (GB 14) and Jingming (BL 1) acupoints to lower border of orbit. Another branch enters ear from Yifeng (TE 17) acupoint and comes out of ear from Ermen (TE 21) acupoint to connect above branch at cheek and then the combined branch goes up to connect foot Shaoyang meridian at Tongziliao (GB 1) acupoint and it further goes to Sizhukong (TE 23) acupoint.

7) Foot Shaoyang gallbladder meridian: The main branch of this meridian originates from Tongziliao (GB 1) beside outer canthus of eye and passes through Shangguan (GB 3) acupoint to Hanyan (GB 4) acu-

point at corner of forehead and then it goes downward behind ear through Fengchi (GB 20) acupoint to neck. A branch enters the ear from the back of ear and comes out of the ear from the front of ear and then it goes to a point behind Tongziliao (GB 1) acupoint and beside outer canthus of eye. Another branch goes downward from Tongziliao (GB 1) acupoint to Daying (ST 5) acupoint to connect hand Shaoyang meridian below orbit. In addition, The main branch of this meridian also goes through face to Muxi (tie of eye) and connects with foot Shaoyang meridian at outer canthus of eye.

8) Foot Jueyin liver meridian: The main branch of this meridian goes upward behind throat to nasopharynx and passes through Daying (ST 5), Dicang (ST 4), Sibai (ST 2) and Yangbai (GB 14) acupoints to directly connect Muxi (tie of eye) and then it comes out from forehead to connect Governor vessel at Baihui (GV 20) acupoint.

In brief, all 3 foot Yang meridians originate from the eye or from the region around eye and 1-2 branches of all 3 hand Yang meridians stop at the eye or the region around eye. In addition, the meridians, branches or main branches of 3 foot Yang meridians, foot Jueyin liver meridian and hand Shaoyang heart meridian are connected to Muxi (tie of eye).

The meridians are densely distributed over the region around the eye to supply sufficient qi and blood to eyes. Therefore, the functional disturbance of meridians may cause diseases of eyes. As mentioned in Miraculous Pivot: The disturbance of hand Yangming large intestine meridian, hand Shaoyin heart meridian, hand Taiyang small intestine meridian and hand Jueyin pericardium meridian may cause yellow color in eyes; the disturbance of foot Taiyang urinary bladder may produce a symptom of eye as if detached from orbit; the disturbance of foot Shaoyin kidney meridian may cause blurred vision; and the disturbance of hand Shaoyang tripple energizer and foot Shaoyang gallbladder meridians may cause pain of outer canthus of eye. As mentioned in The Golden Mirror of Medicine: "The external pathogens may invade the nape to attack Taiyang meridian; invade the face to attack Yangming meridian; and invade the cheek to attack Shaoyang meridian and then the pathogens may be transported through the meridians to the brain to cause diseases of eyes.

(2) Relation between eye and 8 extra meridians

Although the extra meridians are not directly connected with internal organs, they can improve circulation of qi and blood in meridians and enrich supply of nutrients to eyes through the connection with 12 regular meridians. The Dumai (governor vessel), Renmai (conceptional vessel), Yinqiaomai (Yin heel vessel), Yangqiaomai (Yang heel vessel) and Yangweimai (Yang link vessel) among 8 extra meridians are directly connected with eye.

1) Dumai (governor vessel): The Dumai is a meridian to control all Yang meridians in the body and it originates from the center of pubic bone. A branch of Dumai goes up after passing across buttocks to connect foot Taiyang urinary bladder meridian at inner canthus of eye and another branch goes straight upward from lower abdomen, enters throat, passes through lower cheek and stops at a point on the midline of face and below eyes.

2) Renmai (Conceptional vessel): The Renmai is a meridian to control all Yin meridians of the body and it originates from a point below Zhongji (CV 3) acupoint, goes up through abdominal cavity to the lower cheek around the mouth and then travels upward to stop at Chengqi (ST 1) acupoint below eyes after it is split into 2 branches.

3) Yinqiaomai and Yangqiaomai (Yin and Yang heel vessels): The Yin and Yang heel vessels control Yin and Yang on left or right side of body. The Yinqiaomai originates from medial side of heel and goes up to inner canthus of eye to connect Taiyang meridian and Yangqiaomai; and the Yangqiaomai originates from lateral side of heel and goes up to inner canthus of eye to connect Taiyang meridian and Yinqiaomai. The foot Taiyang meridian enters brain from nape and sends out branches to Yin and Yang heel meridians. The Yin and Yang heel meridians connect each other at Jingming (BL 1) acupoint beside inner canthus with qi in them circulating around the eyes to nourish them and control the opening and closure of them. In general, as Weiqi (defensive energy) passing through Yang meridians, the eyes open; and as it passing through Yin meridians, the eyes close. If the qi in Yang heel vessel is excessive and the qi in Yin heel meridian is deficient, the eyes will always open and do not close; and inversely, the eyes will always close and do not open. The invasion of external pathogens may cause redness and pain of eyes and pterygium.

4) Yangweimai (Yang link vessel): The Yangweimai connects all Yang meridians and it originates

from Jinmen (BL 25) acupoint below lateral malleolus and goes upward through lateral and posterior side of lower limb to neck and forehead and then passes through the vertex of head to the occipital region to connect governor vessel. The disease of Yangweimai is an exterior syndrome with headache, red eyes, chillness and fever because all Yang meridians pass through the body surface.

(3) Relation between eye and meridianal muscles

The 12 meridianal muscles are attached to 12 meridians as a group of muscles to control the convergence and divergence of meridianal qi in muscles and joints. Because the meridianal muscles are superficially arranged over the body, they can connect the bones all over the body to control the movement of human body. The meridianal muscles of 3 hand and foot Yang meridians are distributed around the eye.

1) Meridianal muscle of foot Taiyang meridian: A branch of this muscle forms a network above eyes. As explained by Zhang Jingyue: "The muscular network can control the eyelid and eyelash to open and close the eyes."

2) Meridianal muscle of foot Yangming meridian:

A branch of this muscle goes straight upward to face through the side of nose to connect the meridianal muscle of foot Taiyang meridian. It forms a network below eyes to control the opening and closure of eyes in coordination with the muscular network above eyes.

3) Meridianal muscle of foot Shaoyang meridian: The branches of this muscle are distributed around the outer canthus of eye to control the lateral turning of eyeballs.

4) Meridianal muscle of hand Taiyang meridian: The straight branch of this muscle goes up to a point above ear to connect the meridianal muscle of hand Shaoyang and then goes forward and downward to chin to connect the meridianal muscle of hand Yangming meridian. Then it goes upward again to outer canthus of eye to connect the meridianal muscles of hand and foot Shaoyang meridians.

5) Meridianal muscle of hand Shaoyang meridian: A branch of this muscle goes up to Jiache (ST 6) acupoint to meet the meridianal muscle of foot Yangming meridian and then goes up again through the region anterior to ear to connect the meridainal muscles of hand Taiyang and foot Shaoyang meridians beside the outer canthus of eye. Then it goes up to distribute its branch-

es over the corner of forehead.

6) Meridianal muscle of hand Yangming meridian: A branch of this muscle goes up to cheek and distribute branches over cheekbone. A straight branch goes upward along a line anterior to hand Taiyang meridian. The left one goes up through the region anterior to ear to left corner of forehead and send a branch to head, and then it goes down to the right side of chin; and the right branch takes a similar route but on the left side of chin to meet the meridianal muscles of Taiyang and Shaoyang meridians.

All branches and networks of meridianal muscles mentioned above can cooperatively control the opening and closure of eyes, rotation of eyeballs and movement of muscles of head and face. In addition, the meridianal muscle of foot Jueyin liver meridian is also closely related to the eye, because the liver is an organ to control all muscles of the body.

The functional disturbance of meridianal muscles may cause diseases of eyes. As mentioned in Miraculous Pivot: "The diseases of meridianal muscles due to coldness may cause spasm of muscles and opisthotonos; and the diseases due to hotness may cause relaxation and paralysis of muscles." The spasm of left branch of meridianal muscle of foot Shaoyang meridian may cause failure to open right eye and the spasm of right branch may cause failure to open left eye. The diseases of meridianal muscle of foot Yangming meridian due to coldness may cause spasm of muscles and failure to close eyelids; and the diseases due to hotness may cause paralysis of muscles and failure to open eyelids. In addition, the spasm of meridianal muscles of foot Yangming and hand Taiyang meridians may cause deviation of eyes and mouth, spasm of canthi of eyes and sudden blindness. The descriptions in ancient medical books are very useful in the treatment of eye diseases.

(4) Relation between meridians and diseases

The meridian theory is an important component of the basic theories of traditional Chinese medicine as well as a theory of acupuncture and it is very useful in the diagnosis and treatment of diseases. As mentioned by Ma Yuantai, an ancient physician in Ming dynasty: "The diseases may be wrongly diagnosed and treated, if the physicians are not familiar with 12 meridians." The importance of meridians in the diagnosis and treatment of diseases may be illustrated by the following examples:

1) Medical diseases

For diagnosis and treatment of Shanghan (infectious febrile diseases), first of all, the diseases in meridian or in collateral should be differentiated. The patients with diseases in meridian may suffer from headache, stiffness of neck, chillness and floating pulse; if the neck is not stiff, the disease is in collateral rather than in meridian and the drugs for diseases in meridian should not be prescribed to them. The patients with diseases in meridian must suffer from pain in head and nape and stiffness of back, because Taiyang meridian passes upward to Fengfu (GB 20) acupoint in neck.

The patients with diseases in Yangming meridian may suffer from pain in eyes, dryness in nose, inability to lie flat, fever, spontaneous sweating, hatred of hotness instead of coldness and long pulse; if the patients do not suffer from pain in eyes and dryness in nose, it is a disease in collateral rather than in meridian of Yangming, because the Yangming meridian passes along a line beside nose to eyes.

2) Surgical diseases

The sores distributed along Yangming meridian may be quickly cured after putrefaction and healing, because it is rich in qi and blood; the sores along Taiyang and Jueyin meridians may last for a long time and difficult to cure, because they are rich in blood but deficient in qi; and the sores along Shaoyin, Shaoyang and Taiyin meridians are deficult to heal, because they are rich in qi, but difficient in blood. This is a correct way to make prognosis of sores according to the theory about richness of qi and blood in meridians.

The furuncles are usually distributed near the origins or endings of meridians on face, hand and foot. The acupuncture may be applied at the ending (or original) acupoint of a meridian to produce a good result, if the sore is located near the origin (or ending) of that meridian. For example, for a furuncle at Yingxiang (LI 20) acupoint (the last acupoint of large intestine meridian) the acupuncture applied at Shangyang (LI 1) acupoint (the first acupoint of this meridian) may stop pain and reduce WBC count right after the treatment. This is a useful principle for selection of acupoint.

3) Gynaecological diseases

According to the theory of meridian, "the Renmai (conceptional vessel) controls the fetus; and the Chongmai (thoroughfare vessel) controls the reservoir of blood, so that the acupoints of Chongmai can be selected for irregular menstruation and the acupoints of

Renmai are selected for obstetric diseases. The acupoints (or drugs) of stomach, liver and spleen meridians may be selected for the treatment of breast diseases, because they pass through the breast region.

4) Pediatric diseases

The Sifeng (EX-UE 10) acupoints at the creases of first interphalangeal joint of index, middle, ring and little fingers can be selected to treat indigestive malnutrition, because they belong to the large intestine, pericardium, tripple energizers, heart and small intestine meridians.

Before the appearance of poxes, distributed over tripple energizers, the babies may show redness of ear and engorgement of veins behind ear, because the tripple energizer meridian passes through the region behind ear.

5) Application of herbs

As a Yang herb among Yin herbs, Chaihu (Thorowax root) with a slight bitter taste, slight cold nature and ascending effect can produce 4 therapeutic effects: To treat pain in bilateral flanks, tidal fever, blood diseases in internal organs and qi diseases in muscles. Therefore, Chaihu can be used to treat diseases of hand Shaoyang tripple energizer, foot Shaoyang gallbladder, hand Jueyin pericardium and foot Jueyin liver meridians.

2. Relation between eye and internal organs

The eyes can see objects and distinguish colors after the supply of enough nourishment from internal organs to them. As mentioned in Miraculous Pivot: "The essence of internal organs is transported to supply the eyes." It explains the close physiological relationship between eye and internal organs.

(1) Relation between eye and heart and small intestine

1) The heart controls blood and blood vessels and all blood vessels are connected with eyes. As mentioned in Plain Questions: "The blood of whole body is controlled by heart", "the heart is connected with blood vessels", "the blood vessels are the container of blood", and "all blood vessels are connected with eyes." Therefore, the heart can control the blood vessels of the body and promote the circulation of blood through the blood vessels to supply nutrients to eyes for obtaining a good vision.

2) The heart can store spirit and the eyes are the

messenger of heart. As mentioned in Miraculous Pivot: "The eyes are the messenger of heart and the heart is a container of spirit." The mental activity of brain is controlled by heart because the heart is the container of spirit; and the sufficiency of essence in internal organs and condition of mental activity can be shown by the eyes, because they are an external orifice of heart. Therefore, the inspection of eyes is an important method for diagnosis of diseases in traditional Chinese medicine.

3) Relation between eye and small intestine: As mentioned in Miraculous Pivot: "The small intestine is a storage organ in digestion." After digestion is carried out in stomach, the food is transported into small intestine for further digestion and absorption to produce the clear and turbid substances. The clear substance, including the body fluid and nutrients of food and drink, is transported and distributed by spleen to the whole body, including the eyes. The heart and small intestine are a pair of organs with an exterointerior relationship and they are directly connected by meridians. Therefore, the change of function of small intestine can directly affect the heart and indirectly influence the eyes.

(2) Relation between eye and liver and gallbladder

1) The eyes are the external orifice of liver. As mentioned in Miraculous Pivot for discussion of relationship between internal organs and external environment of human body: "The blue is a color of east region in geography and a color of liver in body and the eyes are the external orifice of liver with their essence stored in and supplied from liver. " The nutritive materials stored in liver can be continuously transported to eyes to nourish them.

2) The liver can store blood to improve vision of eyes. The liver can store blood and adjust the amount of blood in body. All internal organs can supply their essence to eyes, but the liver blood is the most important nutrient, becasue the eyes are the orifice of liver. Therefore, a good vision of eyes can be preserved after the liver receives enough blood to store.

3) The liver qi can be transported to eyes. The liver has a dispersing function and it can promote circulation of qi. Qi can produce blood and it can also promote circulation of blood. The supply of blood to eyes always depends on the promotion of qi by liver. As mentioned in Miraculous Pivot: "The liver qi is transported to eyes and then they can distinguish 5 colors, if

the liver function is normal. " Therefore, the eyes can see objects and distinguish colors when the liver qi is rich and well dispersed.

4) The collateral of liver is connected to Muxi (tie of eye) to communicate the internal organs and external structures of body and transport qi and blood to eyes. This is a close linkage between liver and eye in both material supply and functional action.

5) Relation between eye and gallbladder: The liver and gallbladder are a pair of internal organs with an exterointerior relationship and the remaining liver qi is discharged into gallbladder to produce bile after condensation. The bile is very important to eyes. As mentioned in Miraculous of Pivot: "At 50 years of age, the liver is reduced in size, the liver qi becomes deficient and the production of bile is decreased, so that the vision gradually becomes blurred.

(3) Relation between eye and spleen and stomach

1) The spleen can digest food and drinks to produce qi and blood and the essence of spleen is transported to nourish eyes. As mentioned in Plain Questions: "The dysfunction of spleen may cause blockage of orifices of sense organs, anus and opening of urethra."

The eye is one of the 9 orifices and it also depends on the supply of essence from spleen.

2) The spleen has a function to upward spread the clear material, a nutritive product of digestion, to the upper body, including eyes. The eyes can see clear after an enough supply of clear material is distributed by spleen qi.

3) The spleen also has a function to control circulation of blood. The blood vessels are the container of blood and all blood vessels are connected with eyes. The spleen qi can promote the circulation of blood through the vessels in eyes without blood leaking out of the blood vessels and the eyes can see clear after receipt of enough blood supplied by spleen.

4) The spleen can also control muscles to open and close the eyes. The spleen can digest food and drinks to nouish muscles and the muscles of eyelids can freely open and close the eyes after receiving enough nutrients supplied by spleen.

5) Relation between eye and stomach: As a reservoir, the stomach can receive, store and digest food and drinks and the digested food can be transported to small intestine. The nutrients of food obtained after digestion can be distributed by spleen to the whole body. The 9

orifices are controlled by 5 internal organs and the orifices can produce their normal function after the internal organs obtained enough supply of stomach qi, otherwise, the sense organs may lose their normal physiological function.

The spleen and stomach are a pair of internal organs with an exterointerior relationship and they are the fundamental organs to supply essence after birth. The spleen can distribute the clear material upward and the stomach can transport the turbid waste downward. The turbid waste can be discharged from lower orifices, if the spleen and stomach can maintain their normal transporting function. Otherwise, the turbid waste may be adversely sent upward to attack the orifices of sense organs and cause diseases of eyes.

(4) Relation between eye and lung and large intestine

1) The lung is an organ to control qi and the vision is good if qi is moderate. The lungs collect blood from all blood vessels of the body and control qi of whole body. Qi can promote circulation of blood to nourish eyes. The eyes can see clear if the lung qi is moderate, the circulation of qi and blood is smooth, the function of

internal organs is normal to supply enough essence to eyes.

2) The lungs can disperse qi and distribute qi, blood and body fluid to whole body and they can also spread qi downward to transport fluid into urinary bladder. The Weiqi (defensive energy) and body fluid can warm, moist and nourish the eyes if the function of lungs to distribute qi is normal and the blood vessels are patent to preserve the health of eyes.

3) Relation between eye and large intestine: The lung and large intestine are a pair of internal organs with an exterointerior relationship. The waste product of digestion in small intestine is transported to large intestine and then discharged out of the body if lung qi can normally descend to promote discharge of the waste product. Otherwise, the impairment of descending function of lung qi and accumulation of heat pathogen in large intestine may cause diseases of eyes.

(5) Relation between eye and kidney and urinary bladder

1) The eyes can see clear if the kidney essence is sufficient. The essence of human body is a material basis of human life and the good vision of eyes depends on

the nourishment of essence from internal organs, especially from kidney.

2) The kidney can store essence and the essence can produce marrow. The brain is a sea of marrow and the Muxi (tie of eye) is connected with brain. The thought is active and quick and the sight is sharp if the kidney essence is rich and the sea of marrow is full. As proposed by ancient physicians, the eye is a visual organ produced from brain material and it is connected with brain by the cordlike Muxi (tie of eye). Therefore, the image of objects in front of eyes can be projected into the brain through Muxi. This is an explanation of the close relation between eye, brain and kidney.

3) The body fluid is controlled by kidney and it can rinse the eyes. The kidney is an organ to adjust metabolism of water in body and the fluid of internal organs can be transported upward to produce tears for rinsing eyes and to fill the eyeball as Shenshui (miraculous water). The distribution and adjustment of water in eyes as well as in whole body is a function of kidney.

4) Relation of eye and urinary bladder: The kidney and urinary bladder is a pair of internal organs with an exterointerior relationship. In the metabolism of body fluid, the urinary bladder can play a role in tran-

formation of fluid by qi to produce, store and discharge urine. The normal fluid- transforming function of urinary bladder can be maintained in people with sufficient kidney qi and lt may be disturbed to cause retention of body fluid and attack of water and dampness to eyes in people with deficiency of kidney qi or accumulation of damp-heat pathogen in body. In addition, the foot Taiyang is a meridian of urinary bladder to adjust the condition and function of body surface and it may be invaded by external pathogens to cause eye diseases.

(6) Relation between eye and tripple energizer

The tripple energizer is a single internal organ without paired organ and it plays a role in transporting vital energy, water and food and keeping patency of water channel. The essence and fluid supplied to eyes is always transported through tripple energizer. In patients with dysfunction of tripple energizer, the digestion, absorption and distribution of nutrients from food may be disturbed and the eyes can not obtain the nourishment. The blockage of water channel through tripple energizer may cause retention of water in body and eye diseases due to upward attack of water pathogen.

The relation between eye and various internal organs is different in nature and intimacy. The human body is an integrated unit and the eyes have a close physiological and pathological relationship with internal organs through meridians. Therefore, the inspection of eyes is helpful in making diagnosis of diseases.

(7) Introduction of five wheel theory

The eye is divided into 5 wheels (circular zones) from peripheral part of eye to its center and they are related to 5 organs. The upper and lower eyelids are the flesh wheel, related to spleen; the inner and outer canthi are the blood wheel, related to heart; the sclera is the qi wheel, related to lung; the iris is the wind wheel, related to liver; and the pupil is the water wheel, related to kidney.

Following the progress of society, the traditional Chinese medicine has been gradually improved and enriched. In the early Tang dynasty, the etiology of eye diseases, protection of eyes and recipes for eye diseases were already mentioned in the Prescriptions Worth a Thousand Gold for Emergencies and Medical Secrets of an Official published at that time. For example, "the eye diseases may be caused by intake of uncooked, spicy and hot food, indulgence of alcohol or sexual activity and reading books printed with small characters at night ···" However, the 5 wheel theory first appeared in The Peaceful Holy Benevolent Prescriptions written by Wang Huaiyin of Song dynasty in 992.

In Exhaustive and Comprehensive Survey of Silvery Sea, an ophthalmological book published in Song or later dynasty, the theory of 5 wheels and 8 regions was first introduced. As mentioned in this book: "The eye is an important organ to show the essence of 5 internal organs; and the 8 regions are named after 8 Diagrams without defined location."

As mentioned in A Precious Book of Ophthalmology, written by Fu Renyu and published in Ming dynasty: "The 5 wheels can show the essence of 5 internal organs and they are like the turning wheel of vehicle; and 8 regions indicate 8 Diagrams with meridians to connect brain and internal organs and to distribute qi and blood."

The definition of 8 regions was contradictory among different ancient medical books. As mentioned in Exhaustive and Comprehensive Survey of Silvery Sea: "The 8 regions have their names but no definite location." Some ancient physicians believed that the 8 regions are correspondent to 8 Diagrams, but the author of The Golden Mirror of Medicine believed that the 8 regions are correspondent to 6 internal organs.

As mentioned in Essentials of 6 Meridians written by Chen Dafu, a traditional physician in modern times: "The theory of 5 wheels is used to explain the function of different structures of eye; and the theory of 8 regions is used to explain the manifestations of certain diseases of eye. The 8 regions are not necessary to be defined in normal people; and the eye diseases are not all related to 8 regions. Therefore, the theory of 8 regions is seemingly useless in clinical practice, but it should not be rashly abandoned. The theory of 8 regions was first mentioned in the Exhaustive and Comprehensive Survey of Silvery Sea, but the author declared that they have not definite location. The author of The Golden Mirror of Medicine had not mentioned their exact location, although he did not reject the presence of definite locations of 8 regions. The author of A Precious Book of Ophthalmology ascertained the usefullness of this theory in locating the blood streaks in eye diseases and provided a diagram with the names of 4 Diagrams on upper eyelid and the names of another 4 Diagrams on lower eyelid. However, it is too simple to use for clinical practice by the late physicians."

In the Clinical Practice of Traditional Ophthalmology written by Pang Zanxiang, a traditional ophthalmologist in modern times, the author mentioned that the eye is divided into flesh, blood, qi, wind and water wheels from its outer structure to inner structure and they are correspondent to spleen, heart, lung, liver and kidney according to the theory of internal organs. The theory of 5 wheels is used to explain the anatomical, physiological and pathological properties of eye and to guide the diagnosis and treatment of eye diseases.

1) Flesh wheel: It indicates the upper and lower eyelids (including skin, subcutaneous tissues, muscles, tarsal plate and palpebral conjunctiva) closely related to spleen and stomach and it can protect the eyeball. It is named as flesh wheel, because the spleen and stomach can control muscles.

The spleen and stomach are a pair of internal organs with an exterointerior relationship. Therefore, the diseases of flesh wheel are related to the diseases of spleen and stomach. For example, the inflammation of eyelid can be treated with the herbs for clearing damp-heat pathogen in spleen and stomach.

2) Blood wheel: It indicates the blood streaks in inner and outer canthi and the lacrimal caruncle and

lacrimal point in inner canthus for excretion of tears. The blood vessels in both canthi are related to heart and they are called blood wheel, because the heart can control blood. The blood vessels can transport blood and nutrients to nourish eyes.

The heart and small intestine are a pair of internal organs with an exterointerior relationship. The diseases of blood wheel are related to the diseases of heart and small intestine. Therefore, the excessive heat lesions in both canthi can be effectively treated with the herbs to clear fire pathogen in heart.

3) Qi wheel: It indicates the balbar conjuntiva and sclera to protect the internal delicate structures of eye and this is a wheel related to lung, because the lung can control qi.

The lung and large intestine are a pair of internal organs with an exterointerior relationship. The scleral diseases due to heat pathogen in lung may be effectively treated with herbs to clear heat pathogen in lung.

4) Wind wheel: It indicates the cornea and iris. The cornea is a transparent plate with a spherical surface to transmit, condense and reflect light amd the iris is a brownish yellow or brownish black membrane in people of yellow race. The iris can contract and relax to

adjust the light thrown into eyeball for obtaining a clear vision. This wheel is related to liver and the liver can control wind in body. Therefore, it is called wind wheel.

The liver and gallbladder are a pair of internal organs with an exterointerior relationship. The diseases of wind wheel are related to diseases of liver and gallbladder and the keratitis can be treated with the herbs to reduce fire pathogen in liver.

5) Water wheel: It indicates the pupil, but the water wheel actually contains the aqueous humor, lens, vitreous body, choroid, retina and optic nerve. The water wheel is related to kidney and the kidney can control water in body. Therefore, it is called water wheel. The aqueous humor is a transparent liquid filling the anterior and posterior chambers of eye to nourish the lens and vitreous body; the lens is an optic structure with a changeable thickness to reflect light for obtaining a clear image of the object seen by eyes; the vitreous body can both reflect light and maintain the intra-ocular pressure; the choroid is rich in pigment to form a dark chamber as the camera bellows and it also contains rich blood vessels to nourish the retina and nearby structures; the retina is a light-perceiving structure of eye;

and the optic nerve can conduct the information of light, color and figure of visible object into brain. The lesion of any one of above structures may interfere the vision to certain extent.

The kidney and urinary bladder are a pair of internal organs with an exterointerior relationship. Therefore, the optic atrophy can be effectively treated with herbs to tonify kidney.

3. Anatomy of eye

(1) Composition of eye: The eye is composed of eyeball, nerve pathway and accessory structures.

The eyeball is composed of the wall and contents of eye. The wall of eyeball contains 3 layers: the outer layer of cornea, corneal border and sclera; the intermediate layer of iris, ciliary body, choroid and anterior chamber; and the inner layer of retina and the contents of eyeball contain the aqueous humor, lens and vitreous body. The nerve pathway is the afferent nerve and brain. The accessory structures of eye contain the eyelids, lacrimal apparatus, conjunctiva, orbit and extraocular muscles.

(2) Deep structures of eye: There are 8 regions for acupuncture treatment around each eye and the

oblique insertion of acupuncture needle may pierce the skin, superficial and deep fascia to reach orbicular muscles of eye, which should not be pierced through to reach the periosteum.

The superficial fascia at each region contains rich somatic sensory nerves and a network of blood vessels on which are scattered the nerve endings of splanchnic nerve. The inserted needle is wrapped by the network of blood vessels and branches of sensory nerve trunk.

Deep structures in 8 regions: The first region contains the frontal branch of supra-orbital nerve and network of supra-orbital artery; the 2nd region contains the branches of supra-orbital nerve, network of supra-orbital artery and branches of lacrimal nerve; the 3rd region contains the branches of supra-orbital nerve and lacrimal nerve and the network of lacrimal artery, frontal branch of superficial temporal artery and zygomatico-orbital artery; the 4th region contains the palpebral branch of infra-orbital nerve and the network of infra-orbital artery and superficial temporal artery; the 5th region contains the inferior palpebral branch of infra-orbital nerve and the network of infra-orbital artery; the 6th region contains the inferior branch of infra-orbital nerve and infra-orbital artery; the 7th region contains the inferior branch of infra-orbital nerve and infratrochlear nerve and the network of infra-orbital artery and artery of inner canthus; and the 8th region contains the frontal branch of supra-orbital nerve and supratrochlear nerve and the network of supra-orbital artery and frontal artery.

II Division of Eye

The inspection of eye is to observe the shape, color and blood vessels of eye for diagnosis of diseases in internal organs. First of all, the eye should be separated into several divisions to locate and evaluate the change of shape, color and blood vessels of eye and to find the correlation between the abnormal findings of eyes and the disturbance of internal organs.

1. Division of 8 Diagrams

The 8 Diagrams are composed of Qian (乾), Kan (坎), Gen (艮), Zhen (震), Xun (巽), Li (离), Kun (坤) and Dui (兑) Diagrams to indicate 8 natural substances or phenomena, namely the heavens, swamp, fire, thunder, wind, water, mountain and land.

As explained by Yijing (The Book of Changes): The primitive material of universe was divided into Yang (heaven) and Yin (land) through continuous movement and development; again divided into Shaoyang (wood, east or spring), Taiyang (fire, south or summer), Shaoyin (metal, west or autumn) and Taiyin (water, north or winter); and further divided into 8 Diagrams and countless substances and phenomena in the universe. This is a philosophy with a primitive point of view of dialectical materialism.

The theory system of traditional Chinese medicine, including the theory of qi, essence and spirit is derived from the idea of qi (primitive material of the universe), which is composed of Yin qi and Yang qi. All substances and phenomena in the universe can be classified into either Yin or Yang group. For example, the big, thick, white and hot substance, daytime, clear weather and summer season are included in Yang group; and the small, thin, black and cold substance, night, cloudy weather and winter season are included in Yin group. The Yang and Yin substances or phenomena are mutually contradicted and united and this is an idea about the unity of opposites to explain the relationship between all substances and phenomena in the universe. The important principles about differentiation of syndrome for diagnosis and treatment of diseases are all in accordance with the theory of Yin and Yang. All syndromes can be divided into the Yin and Yang categories: The superficial, excessive and hot syndromes are included in the Yang group; and the interior, deficient and cold syndromes are included in the Yin group.

In ancient time, the idea of 8 Diagrams was used for divination. The Confucians used it as a diagram to explain and illustrate the composition and change of the world. The physicians in Song dynasty developed a theory of 5 wheels and 8 regions to explain the physiology, pathology, divisions and clinical manifestations of eye. The 5 wheels are related to 5 internal organs; and the 8 regions are named after 8 Diagrams. This theory produced an important influence on the development of traditional ophthalmology in the following dynasties of China. The sclera is divided into 8 regions according to 8 Diagrams to show the physiological and pathological conditions of different internal organs.

2. Mingmen (life gate) and Sanjiao (triple energizer)

The eye is closely related to internal organs. As proposed by Hua Tuo (an ancient famous physician) in Standards of Diagnosis and Treatment: "In eyes there are 6 large collaterals related to heart, lung, spleen, kidney and Mingmen and 8 medium collaterals related to gallbladder, stomach, large and small intestines, Sanjiao and urinary bladder", and "there are still numerous fine collaterals and small branches". The collaterals (blood vessels) can be seen only on the sclera, but it is too small in area to be divided into 14 zones as the projecting areas of 14 internal organs mentioned above. There are only 12 meridians attached to the internal organs and the Mingmen (life gate) is not included in them, because it is not considered as an internal organ. The Sanjiao is also an organ without a clearcut definition widely accepted. Therefore, the problem of Mingmen and Sanjiao should be discussed first before studying the relation between eye and internal organs.

(1) Mingmen (life gate)

As a gate of life, Mingmen is an important structure to maintain the life of human beings. The kidneys are the paired organs. As mentioned in the Classic on Medical Problems: "The right kidney is called Mingmen and the left one is called kidney", although they are the same in structure and function. This definition is rejected by Yu Bo in his book, Orthodox Medicine and he claimed that Mingmen indicates both kidneys in common rather than the right kidney itself. Some physicians believed that the Mingmen is a source of motive energy located between 2 kidneys, because the Mingmen (GV 4) acupoint is located in a depression below the 2nd lumbar vertebra. Therefore, it is also called the fire of Mingmen. The kidney is a water organ, but it also contains the congenital genuine qi as a fire component in kidney. The congenital genuine qi can be transported upward to combine with the acquired stomach qi for maintaining the life all along.

The functions of Mingmen are as follows:

1) The Mingmen is a source of heat energy and vital qi in human body. 2) It can promote transformation of qi in Sanjiao (triple energizer). 3) The Mingmen fire can warm up spleen and stomach to digest food and drinks.

4) It is closely related to the sexual and reproductive functions of human body and the extraordinary ex-

cessiveness and deficiency of ministerial fire in Mingmen may cause disturbance of above functions.

5) It is closely related to respiration and it can promote inspiration.

(2) Sanjiao (triple energizer)

The Sanjiao is one of the hollow organs and divided into upper, middle and lower energizers. The upper energizer lies above diaphragm and contains heart and lungs; the middle energizer lies between diaphragm and umbilicus and contains spleen and stomach; and the lower energizer lies below umbilicus and contains kidney, urinary bladder and large and small intestines. The function of upper energizer is to distribute fluid and nutrients by heart and lung; the function of middle energizer is to digest and transport food and drinks; and the function of lower energizer is to discharge urine by kidney and urinary bladder and to pass stool from intestine. In brief, the Sanjiao can take in, store and digest food and drinks, produce and distribute qi, blood and nutritive materials and discharge waste products.

The exact anatomical structure and location of Sanjiao is still a problem in dispute. Asmentioned in Miraculous Pivot: "The upper energizer occupies the chest from upper orifice of stomach to throat and it lies above diaphragm; the middle energizer is below upper energizer and contains stomach; and the lower energizer is from ileum to urinary bladder", but the author of Classic in Medical Problems claimed that "Sanjiao has no definite shape". As mentioned by Zhang Jiebin in Illustrative Supplement to Classical Canon: "Xu Dun and Chen Yuanze first declared that the Sanjiao is a piece of omentum as a palm in size and it is in a location opposite to urinary bladder. There are 2 white tubules going up from the omentum along both sides of spinal column to brain". However, Zhang himself believed that "Sanjiao is a protective structure of internal organs. The energizer is red in color with a nature of Yang and fire. The anatomical structures from skin and hair on body surface to internal organs all have their names. What is the name of the big sac filling the whole abdominal cavity? This sac with a red inner lining to protect Yang organs is the triple energizer". As mentioned by Yu Bo in Orthodox Medicine: "Sanjiao is the peritoneal cavity with omentum surrounding the internal organs". In the Correction of Errors in Medicine, Wang Qingren claimed that Sanjiao is the omentum. The omentum was also defined as the triple energizer by Tang Rongchuan in the Treatise in Blood Diseases written by him: "The Shaoyang Sanjiao can command internal organs as the generals command their soldiers and it connects the lungs in upper part and the kidney in lower part of body far away from each other. Therefore, Sanjiao is a big hollow organ without a partner organ and it can control urinary bladder to discharge waste product. As mentioned by Zhang Xichun in the Records of Traditional Chinese Medicine in Combination with Western Medicine: "The Sanjiao, as a circulatory channel of body fluid in western medicine has a pedicle attached to the 11th thoracic vertebra. The upper energizer is a fatty patch below heart; the middle energizer is an omentum wrapping the spleen and stomach; and the lower energizer is an omentum wrapping the kidney and intestines for transportation of fluid into urinary bladder". Following the development of traditional medicine, the anatomy and functions of Sanjiao have been continuously and profoundly studied and it was considered as an important progress of medicine. Five of 6 hollow organs have their partners of 5 solid organs, but Sanjiao is a single hollow organ without a solid organ as its partner. Although the hand Shaoyang Sanjiao and hand Jueyin pericardium are exterointeriorly correlated, they are independent organs. The pericardium as a wall of heart is a part of the heart. Wang Kentang set upper, middle and lower energizers as 3 additional regions on eye and combined them with original 8 regions to locate the projecting areas of internal organs on eye and he again combined the upper energizer with Mingmen as a common region. The author of this book modified Wang's design to locate the projecting areas of internal organs on eye by omitting the Mingmen region and expanding the areas of upper, middle and lower energizer regions.

Upper energizer: The upper energizer occupies the upper part of body above diaphragm and contains the organs in chest, including heart, lungs, trachea, bronchi and pleura as well as the neck, head, face, sense organs and upper limbs.

Middle energizer: It occupies the middle part of body between diaphragm and umbilicus and contains the internal organs in this region, such as liver, gallbladder, pancreas, stomach, intestines and spleen.

Lower energizer: It occupies the lower part of body below umbilicus, including the lumbar, sacral, iliac and hip regions, lower abdomen, urogenital system, anorectal region, peritoneum and lower limbs.

The definition of Sanjiao mentioned above is very helpful in the clinical practice for diagnosis and treatment of diseases.

3. Divisions of eye and relation with internal organs

In order to define 13 projecting areas for 5 solid organs, 5 hollow organs and 3 energizers, the eye is first divided into 8 regions according to 8 Diagrams. The eye can be divided into the upper, lower, left and right parts and the upper and left parts are the Yang regions. First of all, the left eye is divided into 8 regions and defined as 1st, 2nd, 3rd, 4th, 5th, 6th, 7th and 8th regions to take the place of the names of 8 Diagrams.

A horizontal line and a vertical line are drawn across the pupil to divide the eye into 4 quarters and then they are again divided into 8 equal sectors.

For locating 8 regions, the subject is put in a lying flat posture with head toward north. The northwest sector is defined as the 1st (Qian) region of the lung and large intestine (metal organs); the north sector is defined as the 2nd (Kan) region of kidney and urinary bladder (water organs); the northeast sector is defined as the 3rd (Gen) region of upper energizer; the east sector is defined as the 4th (Zhen) region of liver and gallbladder (wood organs); the southeast sector is defined as the 5th (Xun) region of middle energizer; the south sector is defined as the 6th (Li) region of heart and small intestine (fire organs); the southwest sector is defined as the 7th (Kun) region of stomach and spleen (earth organs); and the west sector is defined as the 8th (Dui) region of lower energizer. There is no region on eye for Mingmen and pericardium, because Mingmen is not an organ and the pericardium is a part of heart, but the region for Sanjiao is expanded. The design of projecting areas for internal organs as defined above is very useful in the treatment with eye acupuncture.

How about the arrangement of 8 regions on right eye? The Jing acupoints of 12 meridians are symmetrically arranged on both eyes in a mirror pattern. For example, Chengqi (ST 1) acupoint is directly below the pupils of both eyes; Jingming (BL 1) acupoint is beside the inner canthus of both eyes; and Tongziliao (GB 1) acupoint is beside the outer canthus of both eyes. Therefore, the arrangement of 8 regions or both eyes should also follow this symmetrical relation in mirror pattern.

As concluded by Wang Kentang: "The left eye is a Yang sense organ and the circulation of Yang qi always follows a clockwise pathway, so that the arrangement of 8 regions should also follow this sequence; but the right eye is a Yin sense organ and the circulation of Yin qi always follows a counterclockwise pathway, the arrangement of 8 regions should also follow the reverse sequence".

The distribution of Yin and Yang and the passage of meridians is always symmetrical on both sides of body. Therefore, the arrangement of 8 regions of right eye can not simply copy that of the left eye.

According to the theory of "Yang qi is circulating clockwise and Yin qi is circulating counterclockwise", the arrangement of 8 regions of left eye is in a clockwise sequence and the arrangement of 8 regions of right eye is in a counterclockwise sequence.

The author used this method to inspect eyes and make diagnosis of diseases for more than 10 thousand patients at first visit and obtained a high accuracy of diagnosis. Therefore, this is a new development of inspection of eye for diagnosis of diseases.

After further study, the author of this book again

divided the 8 regions into 13 divisions as the projecting areas of 10 internal organs and 3 energizers. The diagram of 13 divisions of right eye was obtained by turning over that of left eye along a vertical axis. This new diagram of 8 regions and 13 divisions fits in with the principles of passage of meridians and the anatomy of deep structures of eye. The same results of clinical investigation and therapeutic effect of the new diagram have been obtained in comparison with the original diagram.

As mentioned by Li Shizhen in The Study of Eight Extra Meridians about the direct or indirect connection of Yangqiaomai (Yang heel vessel) with inner and outer canthi: "The Yangqiaomai goes upward with foot Yangming meridian to Juliao (ST 3) acupoint, meets Renmai (conceptional vessel) at Chengqi (ST 1) acupoint, joins hand and foot Taiyang meridians, foot Yangming meridian and Yinqiaomai (Yin heel vessel) at Jingming (BL 1) acupoint beside inner canthus, enters hairline from this acupoint, comes out of hair below ear and stops at Fengchi (GB 20) acupoint". As mentioned by Shen Zilu of Ming dynasty in A Complete Book of Meridians: "The outer canthus is a meeting point of hand and foot Shaoyang, triple energizer, gallbladder, hand Taiyang small intestine and foot Taiyang urinary bladder meridians and Yin and Yang heel vessels".

As mentioned by Zhang Jiegu: "The Yin and Yang heel vessels originate from foot and they can play a role in improving the vigorousness and nimbleness of movement of human body. The collateral of Yang heel vessel passes over muscles and through 6 hollow organs to control the structures on body surface; and the collateral of Yin heel vessel passes underneath muscles and through 5 solid organs to control the structures inside the body."

The new diagram of 8 regions and 13 divisions in left eye is same as the original one, but in right eye it is slightly modified. In the new diagram, the liver, gallbladder and upper energizer are close to the outer canthus; and the spleen, stomach and lower energizer are near to the inner canthus. The Yang heel vessel goes upward with foot Yangming meridian and the origin of this meridian is Jingming (ST 1) acupoint just below the 6th (heart and small intestine) region. The Yang heel meridian may also meet the foot Taiyang urinary bladder meridian, so that it is connected with both urinary bladder and kidney, because they are exterointeriorly related. The Yang heel vessel again joins the foot Yangming stomach meridian, therefore, it is also connected with both stomach and spleen. According to the principle of selecting acupoints on the side opposite to lesions, the acupoints of left eye can be used to treat the diseases of both sides. Because the inner and outer canthi of both eyes can connect all internal organs and 3 energizers through Yin and Yang heel vessels, the original and new diagrams can be used to produce a completely equal therapeutic effect and it has been proven by the clinical practice of the author among 3000 patients with various diseases.

4. Remembrance of eye diagram

(1) Remembrance by means of dial plate of clock

The location of 8 regions on sclera can be easily remembered by defining them in terms of a dial plate of clock. Each region occupies a sector of 90 min. The 1st region of left eye occupies a sector from 10:30 to 12:00; the 2nd region from 0:00 to 1:30; the 3rd region from 1:30 to 3:00; the 4th region from 3:00 to 4:30; the 5th region from 4:30 to 6:00; the 6th region from 6:00 to 7:30; the 7th region from 7:30 to 9:00; and the 8th region from 9:00 to 10:30. If the regions are defined by means of the second hand, a sector occupies 7.5 sec and the 1st region is from 52.5 to 60 sec.

The 1st region of right eye occupies a sector reversely from 1:30 to 0:00; the 2nd region reversely from 12:00 to 10:30; the 3rd region reversely from 10:30 to 9:00; the 4th region reversely from 9:00 to 7:30; the 5th region reversely from 7:30 to 6:00; the 6th region reversely from 6:00 to 4:30; the 7th region reversely from 4:30 to 3:00; and the 8th region reversely from 3:00 to 1:30. If defined by second hand, the 1st region is reversely from 7.5 to 0 sec.

(2) Remembrance of projecting areas

The projecting areas of internal organs can be remembered by the pathway of their meridians. As mentioned in Miraculous Pivot: The large intestine and kidney meridians pass beside nostril to a point below eye; the stomach and spleen meridians pass across the nose bridge to a point below eye; the heart meridian connects Muxi (tie of eye); the small intestine meridian stops at inner canthus of eye; the urinary bladder and kidney meridians originate from inner canthus of eye; the triple energizer and pericardium meridians reach outer canthus of eye; the gallbladder meridian originates from outer canthus of eye; the liver meridian connects Muxi (tie of eye), the Dumai (governor vessel) passes through the midpoint between eyes; and the Renmai (conceptional vessel) enters eye.

Besides lung, spleen, kidney and pericardium meridians, 8 of 12 meridians originate from or stop at the eye. The lung, spleen, kidney and pericardium may indirectly connect the eye through their partner meridians. As mentioned in Miraculous Pivot: "The essence of all internal organs can be transported upward to nourish the eye", and as mentioned in Plain Questions: "All meridians are connected with eye". However, the inspection of eye for diagnosis of diseases was first mentioned in the Standards of Diagnosis and Treatment.

As mentioned in above book for easy remembrance of projecting areas of internal organs: The 1st (Qian) region indicates lung and large intestine; the 2nd (Kan) region indicates kidney and urinary bladder; the 3rd (Gen) region indicates upper energizer; the 4th (Zhen) region indicates liver and gallbladder; the 5th (Xun) region indicates middle energizer; the 6th (Li) region indicates heart and small intestine; the 7th (Kun) region indicates spleen and stomach; and the

8th (Dui) region indicates lower energizer.

III Location and Indications of Regions of Eye

The eyeball is divided into 8 regions for diagnosis of diseases.

While looking forward, a vertical and a horizontal lines are drawn through the pupil to divide the eye into 4 quarters and they are further equally divided into 8 sectors as 8 regions of eye.

As mentioned in Plain Questions: "The left and right sides of body are the pathways of Yin and Yang qi", and as explained by Yang Shangshan: "The Yin qi passes through the right side; and the Yang qi through the left side". The right eye is a Yin sense organ with an arrangement of 8 regions in a counterclockwise sequence; and the left eye is a Yang organ with an arrangement of 8 regions in a clockwise sequence. However, the regions on both eyes with a same serial number to represent the same internal organs: The 1st region represents lung and large intestine; the 2nd region represents kidney and urinary bladder; the 3rd region represents upper energizer; the 4th region represents liver and gallbladder; the 5th region represents middle energizer; the 6th region represents heart and small intestine; the 7th region represents spleen and stomach; and the 8th region represents lower energizer.

Each region occupies a sector equal to that of 90 min on the dial plate of clock. For example, the 1st region of left eye is from 10:30 to 12:00 o'clock; and the 1st region of right eye is reversely from 1:30 to 0:00 and by analogy other regions are similarly arranged.

The abnormal manifestations in the regions of eye can show the diseases of their correlative internal organs.

The acupoints of eye are arranged in the orbital region around the eye and one finger width away from the eyeball. The upper border of 8 regions is along a line between the eyebrow and uppereyelid it isand one third from the eyebrow and 2 thirds from the upper eyelid; and the lower border is along a line about 6 − 7 mm below the lower orbital edge. The acupoints of eye are named after the region where they locate. In the 3rd,

5th and 8th regions are the upper, middle and lower energizer acupoints, respectively; and in the 1st, 2nd, 4th, 6th and 7th regions are the lung and large intestine, kidney and urinary bladder, liver and gallbladder, heart and small intestine and spleen and stomach acupoints, respectively. Each of the 5 latter regions is divided into 2 subdivisions for the paired organs and each subdivision occupies a sector of 45 minutes. This arrangement of eye acupoints is known as 8 regions and 13 acupoints.

As mentioned in Classic on Medical Problems, the upper energizer above the diaphragm contains the head, face, sense organs, upper limbs, chest, back, heart, lungs, esophagus and trachea; the middle energizer between diaphragm and umbilicus contains the waist and internal organs in upper abdomen; and the lower energizer below umbilicus contains the lumbar and sacral region, pelvic cavity, hip region, urogenital system and lower limbs.

The 13 acupoints of eye arranged 6.6 mm from the orbital edge have not been mentioned in any ancient and modern acupuncture books. They can produce the same therapeutical effects as 361 body acupoints.

Each eye acupoint can be used to treat the diseases

of its correlated organ:

1. The eye acupuncture can be used to treat the indicative diseases of body acupuncture.

2. The eye acupuncture can produce a good effect to treat hemiplegia caused by cerebral thrombosis, cerebral hemorrhage, cerebral embolism and subarachnoid hemorrhage. The therapeutic effect can be obtained only in patients with a short clinical course within 3 months. The patients with muscular atrophy of shoulder and ilium, failure of arm to flex and difficulty of hand to clench, stiffness or flaccidness of upper and lower limbs and apparent eversion or inversion of foot over half a year should be treated with a combined therapy of eye acupuncture, body acupuncture, physical therapy and administration of traditional and western medicines.

3. The eye acupuncture can produce a good analgesic effect and it can be used to treat headache, toothache, stiff neck with pain, traumatic headache, acute or chronic sprain of wrist and ankle joints, acute colic pain of stomach and intestine, intercostal pain, frozen shoulder, acute cholecystitis, biliary ascariasis, acute orchitis, postoperative pain, acute sprain of waist, neuralgia sciatica, dysmenorrhea, stye and acute

conjunctivitis. For headache due to inflammation, the eye acupuncture can control both pain and inflammation.

4. The eye acupuncture can also be used to treat cutaneous pruritis, gastrointestinal neurosis, insomnia, Parkinson's disease, rheumatic arthritis, cerebral hypoxia due to difficult labor and paralysis of lower limbs due to myelitis.

The sclera in a width of only few cm is divided into 8 regions and 13 acupoints. The areas of 8 regions are the same with each other, but the 1st, 2nd, 4th, 6th and 7th regions are further divided into 2 subdivisions as the projecting areas of lung, large intestine, kidney, urinary bladder, liver, gallbladder, heart, small intestine, spleen and stomach. The eye acupoints are 2mm from the orbital edge and they are very small in area as the tip of finger. Therefore, they should be carefully and accurately located with the center of pupil as a landmark to locate the regions and acupoints.

IV Inspection of Eye for Diagnosis of Diseases

There are many blood vessels on the eyeball. As mentioned by Hua Tuo: "There are 6 large and 8 medium blood vessels in the inner zone and numerous fine blood vessels in the outer zone of eye". The normal blood vessels on conjunctiva are fine and indistinct and the abnormal change of shape and color of blood vessels can be used to make diagnosis of diseases.

1. Change of shape of blood vessels

(1) The expansion of the proximal segments of blood vessels may appear above the level of pupil and it indicates the blood stasis.

(2) The engorgement and varicosis of blood vessels also indicates the blood stasis.

(3) The extension of blood vessels from one region to its nearby region indicates the spread of disease from one organ to another organ.

(4) The branching of blood vessels may appear be-

low the level of pupil and the engorged branches indicate the blood stasis, usually appearing in heart region.

(5) The bulging blood vessels over the bulbar conjunctiva indicate diseases of 6 hollow organs. For example, the bulging blood vessel in large intestine region of left eye indicates hemorrhoids or anal diseases; and the bulging blood vessel in small intestine region indicates the duodenal peptic ulcer.

(6) The ecchymotic patches usually appear in the liver, gallbladder and lower energizer regions and they indicate a depressive syndrome of mind.

(7) The expanding terminals of blood vessels as small beads usually appear in patients with parasites or blood stasis.

2. Change of color of blood vessels

(1) The purplish red blood vessels indicate stagnation of excessive heat pathogen in blood vessels.

(2) The pale blood vessels indicate deficiency of qi and blood or blockage of qi and blood by cold pathogen.

(3) The red blood vessels with black tint indicate the development of an acute disease into heat syndrome; and the change of purple into black color of blood vessels indicates blood stasis caused by excessive

heat pathogen.

(4) The fresh red blood vessels indicate an acute excessive heat syndrome with stagnation of heat pathogen in blood vessels.

(5) The dark grey blood vessels indicate a chronic lesion retained in patients after relief of symptoms.

(6) The dark red blood vessels indicate the deterioration of diseases due to invasion of pathogen from body surface to internal organs or accumulation of heat pathogen in internal organs. The blood vessels of eye are arranged in the superficial and deep layers and the abnormal change of deep blood vessels indicates the diseases of solid organs.

(7) The pale yellow blood vessels indicate the recovery of stomach qi and amelioration of diseases; but the red blood vessels indicate the residual heat pathogen retained in body.

(8) The red blood vessels with yellow tinge indicate the amelioration of disease after the increase of spleen and stomach qi, which is a material basis of life after birth. The yellow is an indicative color of stomach qi.

3. Prognosis by observation of blood vessels

The extension of dark blood vessels from one region to another region indicates the spread of disease to other organ with its primary disease not cured. Otherwise, the primary disease is cured.

The inspection of eye is usually used to diagnose diseases of nervous, cardiovascular and urogenital systems, such as stomach diseases, cholecystitis, biliary ascariasis, hepatitis, indigestion, anal diseases, pain of waist and leg and diseases of head, face and sense organs.

4. Methods of inspection of eye

The patients are asked to relax their eyelids and the physicians may use their clean thumb and index finger to open the eye by pushing the eyelids away from each other. The left eye is observed first and then the right one is observed. The 1st to 5th regions can be first observed when the eyeball is medially turned and then the 6th to 8th regions can be observed when the eyeball is laterally rotated. The inspection of both eyes can be finished within 1 − 2 min without any discomfort born by the patients. The regions with a cluster of blood vessels should be carefully observed.

The findings of inspection of eyes should be drawn on a recording chart or directly written in the medical record of patients.

V Selection of Eye Acupoints

1. Selection of acupoints according to meridians

If the abnormal change of shape and color of blood vessels can be found in the projecting region of the injured organ, the acupuncture applied at this region can produce a good therapeutic result. For example, in patients with acute sprain of waist the fresh red blood vessels may be found in the 2nd region (kidney and urinary bladder) and 8th region (lower energizer) and the acupuncture at those regions may produce a good result.

2. Selection of acupoints according to abnormal change of blood vessels

The region with apparent abnormal change of blood vessels can be selected for treatment of any diseases. For example, the neurotic headache can be cured by the acupuncture treatment applied at 3rd region (upper energizer) of right eye and 4th region (liver and gallbladder) of left eye with apparent abnormal change of blood vessels.

3. Selection of acupoints in Sanjiao regions

The distribution of 3 energizers is expanded in area for the diagnosis of diseases according to inspection of eye. The upper energizer region can be selected for treatment of headache and diseases of upper limb and chest cavity; the middle energizer region is selected for diseases of organs in upper abdomen, back and waist region; and the lower energizer region is selected for diseases of lumbar and sacral region, lower abdomen, urogenital system and lower limb. For example, the acupuncture in 3rd (upper energizer) region of both eyes may produce a good effect to treat frozen shoulder; the acupuncture in 5th (middle energizer) region may produce a good result to treat abdominal pain due to spasm of intestine; and the acupuncture in 8th (lower energizer) region for about 10 min can produce a quick effect to treat acute sprain of ankle joint without fracture of bone and the patients are asked to move their injured joint through the treatment.

4. Localization of acupoints

The exact location of eye acupoints can be determined by pressing the skin in the correspondent region with a probe or the handle of acupuncture needle to find a sensitive spot with a sore, numb, distending, hot, cool, slight pain or comfortable sensation. The sensitive spots can also be located by an electrical detector of meridians and acupoints when the instrument shows the highest peak of electrical current on its scale.

VI Practice of Acupuncture

The acupuncture applied at acupoints near eye may injure the eyeball. Therefore, the eye acupuncture can be performed only by the qualified physician without impairment of vision and tremor of hand and after learning and practice for a long time.

Practice of insertion of needle: After the cover of a square or round box is removed away, a piece of thick and tough paper is glued over the opening of box. Both a closed and an open eye in a real size of human eye are drawn on the paper and 13 eye acupoints in a size of a millet grain are located around the eyes. The open eye is for practice of insertion of needle around the orbital edge; and the closed eye is for practice of insertion of needle into the orbit.

The needle for eye acupuncture is pinched by the thumb and index finger along the direction of the fingers and the needle is inserted exactly into the black spots as the correct location of eye acupoints with one hand when a finger of another hand is put beside the acupoint for fixing and tightening the paper. The insertion of needle should be practised over 1000 times per day and the needle should be inserted vertically, obliquely and horizontally along the subcutaneous tissue. An experienced physician can use both hands to insert needle and it takes about 2 months to learn and practise for mastering a good skill to nimbly and quickly insert needle through the skin by both hands. The paper should be changed every day.

VII Methods of Eye Acupuncture

The stainless steel needle of No. 24 – 32 and 1 cm

in length is gently inserted by one hand when the eyeball is protected and the skin of eyelid is fixed and tightened by the finger of another hand.

The needle should be stably, accurately and quickly inserted. The acupoints for applying acupuncture around the orbit are 2 mm outside the orbital edge. The upper 4 acupoints are along the lower border of eyebrow; and the lower 4 acupoints are along the border between lower eyelid and facial skin. The acupuncture may cause subcutaneous bleeding, if the skin is not tightly fixed while inserting the needle.

The vertical insertion of needle for 3.3 - 6.6 mm may be applied at the sensitive spots; and a horizontal insertion of needle may be applied for 6.6 - 13.2 mm in a projecting region. The vertical insertion is applied with the tip of needle just touching the periosteum; and the horizontal insertion is applied with the tip of needle within the border of a defined projecting region.

The upper, middle and lower energizers occupy a whole region; but other internal organs occupy only one half of a region.

The eye acupuncture may be applied on the diseased side or on the normal side, but a better therapeutic result can be obtained when the eye acupuncture is applied on both sides.

The methods of eye acupuncture can be briefly mentioned as follows:

1. Pricking method: The eye is closed and the eyelid is fixed by a finger. The acupoints are pricked by the tip of needle for 5 – 7 times. This method should be properly applied to avoid causing bleeding of skin. 2. Intra – orbital acupuncture: The needles are vertically inserted around the eyeball toward the orbital wall for 3.3 – 6.6 mm to just touch the periosteum. The insertion of needle does not cause pain if the skin is quickly and smoothly punctured.

3. Horizontal acupuncture: This is an extra – orbital acupuncture and the needles are horizontally inserted for 6.6 – 13.2 mm through the subcutaneous tissue within a defined region.

4. Double acupuncture: Two needles are vertically or horizontally inserted side by side at an acupoint or in a region for enhancing the therapeutic effect.

5. Combined acupuncture: A better therapeutic effect can be obtained by applying both intra – orbital and extra – orbital acupuncture in a same region.

6. Acupressure method: The tip of finger, match and probe or the handle of acupuncture needle can be

used to apply a pressure to the acupoints or regions of eye until a sore or numb sensation is obtained. The patients may be taught to apply this treatment at home for themselves during the attack of pain. It is also very useful for children who are afraid of the puncture of needle.

7. Needle – embedding method: The seeds of cow soapwort or the intradermal needles may be embedded at the acupoints or in the regions for obtaining a prolonged therapeutic effect.

8. Electrical acupuncture: The electrical stimulation may be applied through the needles to the eye acupoints as to the body acupoints, if the simple eye acupuncture alone can not produce any effect after it is applied for 5 min.

9. Contralateral acupuncture: The eye acupuncture may be applied on the eye to the contralateral side of lesion if it can not produce anyeffect as applied on the ipsilateral eye.

10. Combined therapy: The eye accupuncture may be applied alone or in combination with body acupuncture, scalp acupuncture, plum – blossom acupuncture, ear acupuncture, intradermal embedding of needle, massage, Qigong, administration of medicines, water

VIII Needling Sensation and Techniques of Reinforcement and Reduction

After the insertion of needle, it should not be twisted, lifted and thrusted to avoid injuring the eyeball. If a sore, numb, distending, heavy, warm or cool sensation is obtained after insertion of needle, it is an ideal needling response. The needle may be lifted outward for about 1/3 of the depth and inserted again along a new direction if the first insertion has not produced any response. The insertion of double needles or scratching of the handle of needle may be applied for inducing the needling sensation. In patients with a severe disease, chronic disease or paralysis of meridians, the repeated treatment with eye acupuncture may produce certain therapeutic effect, although the acupuncture can not induce any needling sensation.

The horizontal insertion of needle along a direction following the sequence of regions of eye may produce a reinforcing effect; and the insertion of needle along a direction against the sequence of regions may produce a reducing effect.

IX Retention and Removal of Needle

The needle is retained for 5 − 30 min with an average interval of 15 min after the insertion of needle until the symptoms are relieved. Within the period of retention of needle, the handle of needle may be slightly pulled upward or gently twisted within an angle of 10°. The embedding of intradermal needle may be applied to treat some diseases.

For removal of needle, the needle is slowly pulled up by one hand and a piece of sterilized cotton ball is put beside the needle by another hand. The hole of needle is pressed by the cotton ball for a while after the tip of needle is removed off the skin. The needle may be removed by 2 steps, after one half of the needle is pulled out of the skin, it may be held for a few seconds and then the whole needle is removed away with the hole of needle immediately pressed by the cotton ball.

X Cautions

1. The eye acupuncture should be prohibited or carefully performed in patients with swollen eyelids or engorged palpebral veins. It can not be used to treat patients with critical diseases, mental confusion and exhaustion of qi and blood or patients with uncontrollable tremor and restlessness.

2. During insertion of needle, the eyeball should be carefully protected; and after the removal of needle, the orbital edge should be palpated and the patients are asked to open their eyes for ascertaining the safety of treatment.

3. The eyelids should also be protected from injury by eye acupuncture. The needle should not be inserted very deep in the 8th region of both eyes to avoid injuring the artery of inner canthus.

4. The eye acupuncture can be used alone to treat diseases or in combination with administration of medicines for obtaining a better therapeutic effect.

PART 2　TREATMENT OF DISEASES

1. Common cold

The common cold is a common disease caused by external pathogens in 4 seasons, more common in winter, spring and at the time with fluctuation of weather. The chillness, fever, cough and headache are the important symptoms of this disease.

(1) Etiology and pathogenesis

The sweat pores may be obstructed and the lung qi may be blocked by the invasion of wind-cold pathogen to the body surface. The impairment of purifying and descending function of lung due to the attack of wind-heat pathogen to the lungs or the disturbance of defensive function of lung due to the invasion of summer dampness pathogen may also be the causes of this disease.

(2) Differential diagnosis

1) Wind-cold syndrome: The patients may suffer from nasal obstruction, running nose, itching in

throat, cough to spit thin sputum, severe chillness and low fever, no sweating, headache, soreness of limbs, white thin tongue coating and floating tense pulse.

2) Wind-heat syndrome: The patients may suffer from obstruction and dryness of nose with less discharge, sore throat, cough to spit yellow thick sputum, slight chillness, high fever, sweating, headache, thirst, red eyes, yellow thin tongue coating and floating rapid pulse.

3) Summer dampness syndrome: The patients may suffer from heaviness of head as wrapped by a piece of cloth, heaviness, soreness and pain of limbs, low fever, chillness, scanty sweating, mild cough to spit white sticky sputum, chest distress, fullness of upper abdomen, nausea and vomiting, abdominal distension and diarrhea, discharge of a small amount of dark urine, tastelessness and stickiness in mouth, thirst with desire to drink hot water or no thirst, white or yellow greasy tongue coating and moderate or slippery rapid pulse.

(3) Treatment

The No. 32 needles of 3 cm in length are used to do eye acupuncture at lung acupoint in 1st region and upper energizer acupoint in 3rd region. The reinforcing technique by clockwise and horizontal insertion of needle is used to treat the wind-cold syndrome; the reducing technique by counterclockwise insertion of needle is used to treat the wind-heat syndrome; and the reducing technique applied at spleen acupoint in 7th region in addition to above 2 acupoints is used to treat the summer dampness syndrome.

(4) Clinical experience

The similar symptoms may appear in common cold and other infectious diseases at early stage, they should therefore be differentiated from each other. The eye acupuncture is useful to treat common cold. The moxibustion at Zusanli (ST 36) acupoint (3 cun below the lateral depression below patella and one finger width beside the tibial crest) can be applied with moxa cone changed for 3 - 4 times, twice a day to prevent the common cold.

2. Aphonia

This is a symptom with difficulty to produce voice or with hoarse voice to speak and it can be divided into acute and chronic aphonia.

(1) Etiology and pathogenesis

The invasion of external pathogens may block the lung and throat and disturb the function of epiglottis.

In chronic patients the lung and kidney Yin may be exhausted without fluid to moist the vocal apparatus and the purifying and descending function of lung is impaired.

To speak or sing in a loud voice for a long time may injure the vocal apparatus. The mental depression may cause stagnation of qi, transformation of stagnated qi to fire pathogen and coagulation of qi with phlegm to block the vocal apparatus.

(2) Differential diagnosis

1) Acute aphonia: The patients may suffer from sudden hoarseness of voice with itching in throat, cough with sputum, nasal obstruction, running nose, but no thirst; or dryness in nose and throat, cough with yellow sputum, fever, thirst, thin tongue coating and floating tense or floating rapid pulse. Some patients may have normal pulse.

2) Chronic aphonia: The patients may suffer from a gradually worsened hoarseness of voice, leanness of body, dryness in mouth and throat, tidal fever, dry cough, tinnitus, red tongue and thready pulse due to

deficiency of Yin.

The hysterical aphonia with chest distress and belching may be spontaneously relieved.

(3) Treatment

The eye acupuncture is applied at lung acupoint in 1st region and upper energizer acupoint in 3rd region and the kidney acupoint in 2nd region may be added to treat chronic aphonia. The reducing technique is applied to patients with excessive syndrome due to attack of external pathogens or emotional disturbance; and the reinforcing technique is applied to patients with deficient syndrome due to deficiency of lung and kidney Yin or diseases of vocal cord.

(4) Clinical experience

In western medicine the aphonia is caused by acute or chronic laryngitis, small nodules, congestion, swelling and polyps of vocal cord and it may occur in aged patients of cancer. The eye acupuncture applied over a long therapeutic course can produce a good effect on patients with nodules and congestion of vocal cord.

3. Bronchial asthma

The bronchial asthma is a common allergic disease

with repeated relapses. The typical symptom is the paroxysmal attack of dyspnea with wheezing noice.

(1) Etiology and pathogenesis

The impairment of purifying and descending function of lung is caused by the invasion of external pathogens to body surface, accumulation of water or blockage of air passage by phlegm-fire; and the failure of kidney to promote inspiration is caused by deficiency of spleen and wasting of kidney essence.

(2) Differential diagnosis

1) Excessive syndrome: The patients may suffer from severe dyspnea, orthopnea, prolonged expiration, cough with yellow sticky sputum and wheezing noise and the severe patients may even suffer from cyanosis of face and lips, fluttering alae of nose, shrugging shoulders, engorgement of jugular veins, sweating over forehead, annoyance, thirst, constipation to pass dry stool, thin, yellow and greasy tongue coating and slippery rapid pulse.

2) Deficient syndrome: The weak patients with deficiency of kidney may suffer from the similar attack of asthma of excessive type, low coughing voice, spitting of white sputum, hatred of coldness, pale facial complexion, mental tiredness, leanness of body, spon-

taneous sweating, pink or crimson tongue proper with white greasy coating and deep, thready and weak or thready slippery pulse.

(3) Treatment: The lung acupoint in 1st region of eye and Dingchuan (EX-B 1) acupoint of body are used for treatment.

1) Excessive syndrome: The reducing technique is applied at lung acupoint in 1st region, spleen and stomach acupoints in 7th region of eye and Dingchuan (EX-B 1) acupoint of body for dispersing qi of lung and resolving sputum.

2) Deficient syndrome: The reinforcing technique is applied at lung acupoint in 1st region and kidney acupoint in 2nd region of eye and Dingchuan (EX-B 1) and Zusanli (ST 36) acupoints of body for tonifying kidney, promoting inspiration and improving body resistance.

(4) Clinical experience

The eye acupuncture can produce a good immediate and remote therapeutic effect and the cupping therapy at back Shu acupoints can control asthma due to cold pathogen. The patients should maintain their body warmth, prevent common cold, perform physical exercise to improve body resistance. The sea food and allergic and irritative food are prohibited.

4. Cough

The cough with coughing noise and spitting of sputum is a common symptom of respiratory diseases. The acute cough is due to the attack of external pathogens and the chronic cough caused by damage of internal organs is often accompanied with asthma.

(1) Etiology and pathogenesis

The exccessive cough is due to impairment of dispersing function of lung and upward rushing of lung qi caused by invasion and accumulation of external pathogen in lung. The cough may also be caused by disturbance of internal organs, including the scorching of lung and stomach the fire pathogen derived from greasy and spicy food overeatten by the patients; the production and upward attack of phlegm and dampness pathogen to the lung in patients with impaired digestive function of spleen; and the transformation and upward attack of fire pathogen derived from stagnated liver qi along the meridian to lungs in patients with mental depression.

(2) Differential diagnosis

1) Cough due to wind-cold pathogen: The patients may suffer from cough with loud coughing voice, itching in throat, spitting of white thin sputum, chillness, fever, no sweating, headache, nasal obstruction with running nose, soreness of limbs, white thin tongue coating and floating or floating tense pulse.

2) Cough due to wind-heat pathogen: The patients may suffer from repeated cough with loud noise and sticky or yellow sticky sputum difficult to spit out, pain and dryness in throat, fever, chillness induced by blowing wind, slight sweating, headache, turbid nasal discharge, yellow thin tongue coating and floating rapid pulse.

3) Cough due to deficiency of lung: The patients may suffer from cough with low coughing voice, weakness, shortness of breath induced by slight physical exertion, spitting of white, clear and thin sputum, mental tiredness, no desire to speak, pale complexion, chillness induced by blowing wind, spontaneous sweating, susceptibility to common cold, white tongue coating and thready weak pulse.

4) Cough due to phlegm and dampness pathogen: The patients may suffer from cough in the morning

with loud coughing voice and profuse sticky sputum, relief of cough after evacuation of sputum, chest distress, poor appetite, tiredness of body, white greasy tongue coating and soft slippery pulse.

5) Cough due to liver fire pathogen: The patients may suffer from repeated cough with shortness of breath and flushing face caused by emotional distrubance, pain in chest and flanks caused by cough, bitter taste in mouth, spitting of scanty sticky sputum firmly attached to throat, red tip of tongue, yellow thin coating and stringy rapid pulse.

(3) Treatment: To expel wind-cold or wind-heat pathogen, disperse lung qi or clear heat in lung, control cough and resolve sputum.

1) Excessive cough due to attack of external pathogens: The reducing technique is applied at acupoints selected by inspection of blood vessels on eye with the needles immediately removed or retained for 5 – 15 min, once or twice a day.

2) Deficient cough or mixed type of excessive and deficient cough due to injury of internal organs: The reinforcing technique or even reinforcing and reducing technique is applied at kidney acupoint in 2nd region for cough due to deficiency of lung; at spleen acupoint in

7th region for cough due to phlegm and dampness pathogen; and at liver acupoint in 4th region for cough due to liver fire pathogen, once a day during the attack of cough and 2 – 3 times a week after the relief of cough.

(4) Clinical experience

The eye acupuncture can produce a good therapeutic effect to control cough. If it is ineffective in chronic cough, a combined therapy may be adopted to treat the patients. The patients should perform physical exercise to improve their body resistance, keep the body warmth and avoid eating spicy and greasy food, smoking cigarettes and overfatigue. The patients of chronic cough refractory to the conservative treatment should receive a thorough examination to rule out the serious organic lesions in lung and trachea.

5. Vomiting

The vomiting is a common symptom occurring in many acute and chronic diseases with contents in stomach vomited out of the mouth.

(1) Etiology and pathogenesis

1) Acute vomiting: The acute vomiting is due to

attack of external pathogens to stomach, inadequate diet and stagnation of food in stomach or loss of regulating and descending function of stomach caused by emotional disturbance or adverse attack of stagnated liver qi to stomach.

2) Chronic vomiting: The chronic vomiting in patients with a chronic disease and deficiency of qi is due to reduction of stomach and spleen Yang qi and impairment of digestive function, production and accumulation of phlegm and rheum in stomach and adverse ascent of stomach qi.

(2) Differential diagnosis

1) Attack of external pathogens: The patients may suffer from sudden onset of vomiting, distress in chest and upper abdomen, chillness, fever, headache, soreness of limbs, white thin tongue coating and floating pulse.

2) Stagnation of food: The patients may suffer from regurgitation of sour and putrefied food debris, distension of upper abdomen, poor appetite, belching, relief of symptoms after vomiting, constipation or diarrhea, thick greasy tongue coating and slippery strong pulse.

3) Stagnation of phlegm and rheum: The patients

may suffer from vomiting of sputum and saliva, distress in chest and upper abdomen, poor appetite, dizziness, palpitation of heart, white greasy tongue coating and slippery pulse.

4) Stagnation of liver qi: The patients may suffer from regurgitation of sour fluid, pain and distension in upper abdomen and flanks, repeated belching, aggravation of symptoms by mental depression, red borders of tongue proper, thin greasy or yellow coating and stringy pulse.

5) Weakness of spleen and stomach: The patients may suffer from vomiting from time to time after overeating of food or overfatigue, poor appetite, mental and physical tiredness, diarrhea, pale tongue proper and soft weak pulse.

(3) Treatment: To adjust stomach and control vomiting.

The reducing technique of eye acupuncture is applied at middle energizer acupoint in 3rd region and stomach acupoint in 7th region for excessive syndrome; reinforcing technique for deficient syndrome; and even reducing and reinforcing technique for cold and deficient syndrome due to accumulation of phlegm and rheum.

(4) Clinical experience

The eye acupuncture can produce an apparent effect to treat vomiting of various causes, and it is especially useful to control the acute vomiting. For obtaining a better result, the causes of vomiting should be carefully evaluated, because the eye acupuncture can only produce a temporary relief in patients with vomiting due to cancer or diseases of brain.

The patients with vomiting due to chronic diseases of stomach should be on a proper diet regime without cold and uncooked food and they should keep a pleasant mood.

6. Hiccup

The hiccup is a symptom with air suddenly and automatically rushing out of throat to produce a noise and it may appear alone without other symptoms or in many acute and chronic diseases.

(1) Etiology and pathogenesis

The hiccup may be caused by overeating of cold and uncooked food and accumulation of cold pathogen in stomach; by overeating of spicy food and accumulation of heat pathogen in stomach; by adverse attack of stagnated liver qi to stomach; and by loss of regulating and descending function of stomach due to deficiency of spleen and stomach Yang or deficiency of stomach Yin.

(2) Differential diagnosis

1) Stomach cold type: The patients may suffer from slow hiccup with a low voice, aggravation of hiccup by coldness and alleviation by hotness, pain and cold feeling in upper abdomen, poor appetite, white thin tongue coating and slow moderate pulse.

2) Stomach heat type: The patients may suffer from rushing hiccup with a loud noise, annoyance, foul smell from mouth, thirst with desire to drink cold water, discharge of dark urine in short stream, constipation, red tongue proper with yellow coating and slippery rapid pulse.

3) Qi stagnation type: The patients may suffer from hiccup related to emotional disturbance, chest distress, belching, distension of upper abdomen and flanks, white thin tongue coating and stringy pulse.

4) Yang deficiency type: The patients may suffer from hiccup with a low and weak noise, shortness of breath, pale facial complexion, cold limbs, reduced intake of food, tiredness, diarrhea, pale tongue proper with white coating and thready weak pulse.

5) Yin deficiency type: The patients may suffer

from short intermittent hiccup, dryness of tongue and mouth cavity, extreme thirst, annoyance, red tongue proper with scanty coating and thready rapid pulse.

(3) Treatment

The patients are asked to close their eyes and after the local skin is sterilized, the eyeball is pressed by a finger of the physician to tighten the skin of eyelids for horizontal insertion of a No. 32 needle of 1.5 cm in length at upper energizer acupoint in 3rd region, middle energizer acupoint in 5th region and spleen and stomach acupoints in 7th region, 6 - 7 mm from the orbital edge. The needles are retained for 15 - 20 min after the needling sensation is obtained and the treatment may be applied 1 - 2 times a day.

(4) Clinical experience

The eye acupuncture can produce a good result to treat hiccup in patients with excessive syndrome, but its therapeutic effect is poor in deficient syndrome. The appearance of hiccup in critical patients indicates a bad prognosis.

The temporary hiccup due to attack of cold weather or quick swallowing of food can be controlled soon after heavily pressing bilateral Cuanzhu (BL 2) acupoints together with deep breath, sneezing induced by stimulating nasal mucosa and drinking of hot water.

7. Stomachache

The stomachache is a common symptom of acute or chronic gastritis, gastric and duodenal peptic ulcer, gastric neurosis, stomach cancer, ptosis of stomach and some diseases of liver and gallbladder with pain in upper abdomen.

(1) Etiology and pathogenesis

The stomachache may be caused by injury of spleen and stomach and dysfunction of stomach due to improper diet regime, extreme hunger or fullness, indulgence of delicious food and overeating of cold and uncooked food; by adverse attack of stagnated liver qi to stomach due to emotional disturbance, fury or mental depression and the wasting of stomach Yin and poor nourishment of stomach due to transformation of stagnated liver qi to fire pathogen to scorch the collaterals of stomach; by loss of regulating and descending function of stomach due to attack of both external and internal cold pathogen and reduction of spleen and stomach Yang; or by damage of collaterals of stomach in patients with longstanding stomachache to produce bleeding in stomach.

(2) Differential diagnosis

1) Stagnation of liver and stomach qi: The patients may suffer from epigastric distension and pain radiated to flanks and exacerbated by mental depression, belching, regurgitation of sour fluid, poor appetite, thin tongue coating and stringy pulse.

2) Flaming of fire in stomach: The patients may suffer from severe burning pain in epigastric region, dryness and bitter taste in mouth, regurgitation of sour fluid, heartburn, restlessness, anger, red tongue proper with yellow coating and stringy rapid pulse.

3) Food injury of spleen and stomach: The patients may suffer from distension and pain in epigastric region, anorexia, foul smell from mouth, belching and regurgitation of sour and putrefied fluid, vomiting or diarrhea, thick and greasy tongue coating and slippery pulse.

4) Blood stasis in stomach: The patients may suffer from repeated relapses of pricking or cutting pain in epigastric region without fixed location for a long time, hatred of local palpation, vomiting of blood, passage of bloody stool, dark purple tongue proper and uneven

pulse.

5) Deficiency and coldness of spleen and stomach: The patients may suffer from dull pain in epigastric region, preference for hotness and palpation, regurgitation of clear fluid, cold limbs, mental tiredness, diarrhea, pale tongue proper with white thin coating and thready weak pulse.

6) Deficiency of stomach Yin: The patients may suffer from pain and hotness in epigastric region, hunger without desire to take food, thirst without desire to drink water, hot sensation in palms and soles, constipation, red tongue proper with scanty coating and thready pulse.

(3) Treatment: To adjust stomach qi.

The reducing technique is applied for excessive syndrome and the reinforcing technique applied for deficient syndrome at stomach acupoint in 7th region, middle energizer acupoint in 5th region and other eye acupoints according to the inspection of blood vessels on eyes. (4) Clinical experience

The eye acupuncture can produce an analgesic effect to control stomachache of different types and it may produce a good effect to treat acute spasm of stomach. The persistent application of eye acupuncture can resolve the inflammation and promote the healing of ulcer in stomach. The moxibustion at Zusanli (ST 36) and Qihai (CV 6, 1.5 cun below umbilicus) acupoints is useful to treat the patients of peptic ulcer with a short clinical course, in remission stage and without severe complications.

Through the therapeutic course, the patients should take the digestible food and avoid eating the cold and uncooked food. They should keep a pleasant mood and protect their stomach from the attack of coldness.

8. Jaundice

The jaundice is a symptom of many diseases with yellow eyes, skin and urine.

(1) Etiology and pathogenesis

The external damp-heat and epidemic toxic pathogens after invading the body may be accumulated in Zhongjiao (middle energizer) to block the discharge of bile, which may be spread to skin, muscles and urinary bladder to stain the eyes, skin and urine; and the jaundice may also be caused by accumulation of endogenous dampness pathogen in patients with impairment of digestive function of spleen to block the discharge of bile.

(2) Differential diagnosis: The jaundice can be divided into Yang and Yin types according to the clinical manifestations of patients and pathological processes of diseases.

1) Yang type of jaundice: The patients may suffer from fresh yellow eyes and skin in orange color, fever, dryness in mouth, thirst with desire to drink cold water, distension of abdomen, anguished feeling in heart, discharge of dark urine in short stream, constipation, yellow greasy tongue coating and stringy rapid pulse. The patients with invasion of toxic-heat pathogen may suffer from mental confusion, skin rashes and cutaneous hemorrhage; and the patients with dominance of dampness over heat pathogen may suffer from dull yellow skin, low fever, fullness of epigastric region, diarrhea, no thirst and soft rapid pulse.

2) Yin type of jaundice: The patients may suffer from dark and smoky yellow eyes and skin, mental tiredness, hatred of coldness, reduction of intake of food, fullness of epigastric region, soft stool, tastelessness in mouth, no thirst, pale tongue proper with greasy coating and soft or deep slow pulse. The patients of jaundice with blood stasis and abdominal masses may

suffer from pain and distension in subcostal region, leanness of body and distension of abdomen, marked reduction of food intake, purple tongue proper with ecchymoses and thready uneven pulse to indicate the presence of malignancy.

(3) Treatment: The reducing technique is applied for Yang jaundice and the even reinforcing and reducing technique is applied for Yin jaundice at bilateral liver and gallbladder acupoints in 4th region, spleen acupoint in 7th region and middle energizer acupoint in 5th region and the needles are retained for 20 min, once a day. A therapeutic course lasts for 10 days and a rest for 3 days is arranged between 2 courses.

(4) Clinical experience

The eye acupuncture can produce an apparent effect to treat hepatocellular and obstructive jaundice and it is especially useful to treat acute icteric viral hepatitis. The patients with obstructive jaundice should be carefully observed during the conservative therapy for not losing the change of surgical intervention; and the patients with subcostal masses should be examined to rule out the presence of malignancy.

9. Cholelithiasis

This is a disease with stone or sand present in biliary tract and in traditional Chinese medicine it is included in the diseases of pain in flank, jaundice or epigastric pain.

(1) Etiology and pathogenesis

The formation of sand and stone in biliary tract is due to stasis of liver and gallbladder qi, stagnation of damp-heat pathogen, accumulation of bile and transformation of stagnated liver qi into fire pathogen.

The jaundice is caused by blockage and overflow of bile due to stagnation of liver qi and dysfunction of spleen and stomach.

(2) Differential diagnosis

1) Qi stagnation type: The patients may suffer from persistent distending or colic pain in right upper quadrant of abdomen induced by emotional disturbance or intake of oily food, poor appetite, belching, nausea, vomiting, low fever or no fever, local tenderness, white thin or yellow, thin and greasy tongue coating and stringy, tense and rapid pulse.

2) Damp-heat type: The patients may suffer from distending or severe colic pain in right upper quadrant of abdomen, bitter taste in mouth, poor appetite, distress in chest and abdomen, nausea, vomiting, chillness, fever, occasional jaundice of eyes and skin, yellow greasy tongue coating and stringy slippery pulse.

(3) Treatment

The eye acupuncture is applied at bilateral liver and gallbladder acupoints in 4th region and middle energizer acupoint in 5th region. The needles are inserted clockwise in left eye and counterclockwise in right eye and retained for 5 min.

(4) Clinical experience

The therapeutic effect of electrical acupuncture is better than that of pure acupuncture. In patients with sudden exacerbation of abdominal pain during the treatment, the eye acupuncture may be continued, if they have not high fever and symptoms of intoxication, because it may be an indicative sign of spontaneous discharge of stone. The sudden relief of symptoms is an indication of discharge of stone, but it is not remarkable in the discharge of small stone and sand. The stone over 1 cm in diameter is difficult to be spontaneously discharged and the sand can not be completely discharged.

10. Abdominal pain

The abdominal pain is a common symptom occurring in many diseases, but only the abdominal pain caused by invasion of external pathogens, improper diet, emotional disturbance and deficiency of Yang of internal organs will be discussed as follows. The acute and chronic enteritis, intestinal spasm and intestinal neurosis in western medicine can be effectively treated by eye acupuncture accordingly.

(1) Etiology and pathogenesis

The cold pathogen may be accumulated in body after the invasion of external cold pathogen or intake of cold and uncooked food to block circulation of qi and disturb the digestion; the improper diet or overeating of food may cause indigestion, accumulation of food and stagnation of heat pathogen to block transportation of stomach and intestine; the emotional disturbance may cause stagnation of liver qi, accumulation of qi and blood and dysfunction of liver and stomach; and the reduction of spleen Yang in patients with general deficiency of Yang in the past may cause stagnation of cold and dampness pathogens and impairment of digestion.

(2) Differential diagnosis

1) Invasion of cold pathogen: The patients may suffer from severe abdominal pain aggravated by coldness and alleviated by hotness, no thirst, diarrhea, discharge of clear urine, white thin tongue coating and deep tense pulse.

2) Stagnation of food: The patients may suffer from pain and distension of abdomen, anorexia, regurgitation of sour and putrefied fluid, tenderness of abdomen and hatred of palpation, induction of defecation by pain and relief of pain after defecation, greasy tongue coating and slippery pulse.

3) Stagnation of qi: The patients may suffer from wandering abdominal pain induced by emotional disturbance and radiated to flanks, bitter taste in mouth, white thin tongue coating and stringy pulse.

4) Deficient cold syndrome: The patients may suffer from intermittent dull pain of abdomen, preference for hotness and pressure, diarrhea, mental tiredness, hatred of coldness, pale tongue proper with white coating and deep thready pulse.

(3) Treatment

The reducing technique of eye acupuncture is applied at upper energizer acupoint in 3rd region, middle energizer acupoint in 5th region and other acupoints of both eyes according to the inspection of blood vessels on eye for abdominal pain due to attack of cold pathogen; the even reinforcing and reducing technique for abdominal pain due to stagnation of qi; and the reinforcing technique for deficient cold syndrome.

(4) Clinical experience

The eye acupuncture can produce a good effect to control pain of abdomen in acute and chronic enteritis and intestinal spasm. The abdominal pain in patients of acute abdomen may be relieved by electrical acupuncture, but the patients should be carefully observed for not losing the chance of surgical intervention.

11. Diarrhea

The diarrhea is a symptom of acute and chronic enteritis, intestinal tuberculosis and intestinal dysfunction to pass loose or watery stool for many times in a day and it is common in summer and autumn season.

(1) Etiology and pathogenesis

The invasion of external cold dampness or damp-heat (of summer) pathogen may injure spleen and stomach and disturb the function to transport food and to separate clear and turbid products of digestion; the overeating of cold, uncooked and greasy food or intake of unhealthy and contaminated food may injure stomach and intestine and cause impairment of digestion; the worriment and anger over a long time may cause stagnation of liver qi and dysfunction of spleen; and the patients with weak spleen and stomach in the past may develop impairment of digestion and blockage of clear qi to descend. The kidney may also be involved in chronic patients to cause loss of warmth from spleen and stomach and poor digestion of food and drinks.

(2) Differential diagnosis

1) Cold dampness type: The patients may suffer from urgent defecation of watery stool, abdominal pain, increase of intestinal gurgles, distress in upper abdomen, reduction of food intake; or chillness, fever, headache, pain in body, white slippery or white thin tongue coating and floating tense pulse.

2) Damp-heat type: The patients may suffer from prompt passage of yellowish brown, foul and watery stool, abdominal pain, burning pain of anus, hot sensation and annoyance in heart, thirst, discharge of dark urine in short stream, yellow greasy tongue coating and

slippery rapid pulse.

3) Food injury type: The patients may suffer from diarrhea with foul stool, abdominal distension and pain relievable after defecation, poor appetite, regurgitation of sour and foul fluid, dirty tongue coating and slippery forceful pulse.

4) Spleen deficiency type: The patients may suffer from chronic intermittent diarrhea with indigested food induced by improper diet and careless living, abdominal distension, intestinal gurgles, poor appetite, sallow complexion, mental tiredness, pale tongue proper with white coating and thready weak pulse.

5) Kidney deficiency type: The patients may suffer from diarrhea in early morning with indigestive food in feces after intestinal gurgles, cold limbs and body, soreness of waist, weakness of knees, pale tongue proper with white coating and deep thready pulse.

6) Liver stagnation type: The patients may suffer from diarrhea after abdominal pain and related to emotional disturbance, relief of abdominal pain after defecation, repeated flatus, belching, reduction of food intake, white thin tongue coating and stringy pulse.

(3) Treatment

The eye acupuncture is applied at large intestine

acupoint in 1st region. The lung acupoint in 1st region and spleen acupoint in 7th region may be added to expel superficial pathogens and eliminate dampness for patients of diarrhea caused by external pathogens; the spleen and stomach acupoints in 7th region may be added to promote digestion for patients with diarrhea due to food injury; the kidney acupoint in 2nd region and spleen acupoint in 7th region may be added to improve body resistance for patients with chronic diarrhea; the kidney acupoint in 2nd region and middle energizer acupoint in 5th region may be added to warm kidney and arrest diarrhea for patients with deficiency of kidney; and the liver acupoint in 4th region can be added to disperse liver qi for patients with diarrhea due to stagnation of liver qi.

(4) Clinical experience

The eye acupuncture can produce an apparent effect to treat diarrhea, but it can only relieve the symptoms for patients of chronic leukemia, pulmonary heart disease or organic lesions in digestive tract with diarrhea. The patients of diarrhea with severe dehydration should be treated with intravenous infusion of fluid. The food hygiene, proper diet regime and maintenance of body warmth is also important for prevention of diarrhea.

12. Constipation

The constipation is a symptom to pass dry and hard stool once over several days and it can be divided into excessive and deficient types.

(1) Etiology and pathogenesis

The excessive constipation may be caused by accumulation of heat pathogen in stomach and intestine due to overeating of spicy and fried food or exhaustion of fluid in intestine due to attack of warm and heat pathogen in patients with excessive Yang in the past; and the deficient constipation is caused by accumulation of cold pathogen in intestine of aged patients with deficiency of essence in lower energizer; or caused by deficiency of qi and blood to nourish and moisten the intestine after chronic diseases or delivery of baby.

(2) Differential diagnosis

1) Excessive constipation: The patients may suffer from constipation, abdominal distension, hatred of hotness and preference for coldness, dryness in mouth to drink much water, passage of dark urine, red tongue

proper with yellow dry coating and full rapid pulse.

2) Deficient constipation: The patients may suffer from constipation due to weak evacuating force of intestine, weakness of body, mental fatigue, sallow complexion, dizziness, palpitation of heart, frequent discharge of urine, coldness below waist, pale tongue proper with thin coating and deep thready pulse.

(3) Treatment

The patients are asked to close their eyes and after local sterilization of skin, the eyelid is pressed by a finger of the physician to tighten the skin for horizontal insertion of No. 32 needles of 1.5 cm in length 6 mm from the orbital edge and the needles are retained for 15 - 20 min, once a day. The reducing technique is applied to patients with excessive constipation and the reinforcing technique is applied with moxibustion at Mingmen (GV 4, in a depression below L2 vertebra) and Qihai (CV 6) acupoints for deficient constipation in patients with cold feeling below waist.

(4) Clinical experience

The eye acupuncture can produce an apparent effect to treat constipation. The intake of more vegetables and abdominal massage are useful to treat habitual constipation.

13. Prolapse of rectum

This is a disease with rectum, anal canal and even distal end of sigmoid colon dropped out of anus and it is common in aged people, children and multiparous women.

(1) Etiology and pathogenesis

The prolapse of rectum may be caused by deficiency of spleen and kidney after chronic diarrhea or dysentery in weak patients; by exhaustion of vital energy after child birth in multiparous women; by exhaustion of essence in lower energizer, descent of qi of middle energizer and failure to hold the organs in their normal position in patients with chronic cough and constipation; or by accumulation of damp-heat pathogen due to indulgence of greasy and delicious food to imperil the controlling function of anus.

(2) Differential diagnosis

1) Qi descent type: The patients may suffer from prolapse of rectum after bowel movement, heavy physical exertion or severe cough, but no local redness, swelling, hotness and pain. The rectum can be put back only by manual replacement. At the same time,

they also have symptoms of mental tiredness, physical weakness, pale face and lips, poor appetite, pale tongue proper with white thin coating and thready weak pulse.

2) Damp-heat type: The patients may suffer from prolapse of rectum with local redness, swelling, hotness and pain at the early stage of dysentery or during the attack of hemorrhoid with inflammation and constipation, dryness of tongue and oral cavity, red tongue proper with yellow coating and stringy rapid pulse.

(3) Treatment

The reinforcing technique of eye acupuncture is applied at large intestine acupoint in 1st region, lower energizer acupoint in 8th region and other acupoints according to the inspection of blood vessels on eye for patients with prolapse of rectum of deficient type; and the reinforcing technique with moxibustion at Baihui (GV 20, on the vertex of head and at the midpoint between bilateral apexes of ear) acupoint for deficient type. The acupuncture needle of 4.5 - 7.5 cm in length is used to do body acupuncture at Changqiang (GV 1, below the tip of coccyx) acupoint to produce a needling sensation spread around the anus by a twisting technique.

(4) Clinical experience

The eye acupuncture is useful to replace the prolaptic rectum, although it can not cure this disease. The prolaptic rectum must be put back by manual replacement right after bowel movement to prevent the strangulation of rectum, if it can not be replaced spontaneously. The external drugs should be applied to patients of this disease with local redness, swelling and ulceration. The patients should perform physical exercise for improving their health and establish a habit of regular bowel movement.

14. Hypertensive disease

This is a chronic general disease with an increased arterial blood pressure and it is included in the disease of liver Yang, liver fire or vertigo in traditional Chinese medicine.

(1) Etiology and pathogenesis

This disease is caused by flaming up of liver fire and transformation of excessive fire into wind pathogen due to overeating of sweet and greasy food to produce much phlegm and dampness pathogen as well as overeating of spicy food, indulgence of alcohol, emotional disturbance and angry; or caused by insufficiency of kidney water to moisten liver and hyperactivity of liver Yang in people with excessive sexual activity or in aged people.

(2) Differential diagnosis

1) Ascendant hyperactive liver Yang type: The patients may suffer from pain and distention of head, dizziness, blurred vision, hotness of face, high irritability, dryness in mouth, discharge of dark urine, yellow thin or yellow dry tongue coating and stringy slippery pulse.

2) Yin deficiency and Yang hyperactivity type: The patients may suffer from headache, vertigo, blurred vision, dryness in mouth, flushed face or tinnitus, palpitation of heart, insomnia, numbness in limbs, red or crimson tongue proper with yellow thin coating or exfoliated tongue and stringy thready pulse.

(3) Treatment

The liver acupoint in 4th region is selected for applying eye acupuncture to produce an apparent hypotensive effect. The upper energizer acupoint in 3rd region is added to calm liver and subdue Yang for the first type; and the kidney acupoint in 2nd region is added to tonify kidney and drain pathogen from liver for the second type.

(4) Clinical experience

The eye acupuncture can produce an apparent effect to treat essential hypertension of stage I and stage II, but the patients of stage III should be treated with a combined therapy. For treatment of secondary hypertension the causes of disease should be eliminated. The alcohol and spicy food are prohibited to take.

15. Palpitation of heart

This is a subjective symptom with a distressing and unstable sensation in heart and it can be divided into Jingji (frightening) and Zhengchong (continuous violent beats of heart). The patients of various heart diseases, cardiac valvular diseases, myocarditis, cardiac arrhythmia or neurasthenia with palpitation of heart can be treated by the following methods.

(1) Etiology and pathogenesis

The palpitation of heart is usually caused by emotional disturbance or invasion of external pathogens in people with a weak physique. This symptom may be caused by deficiency of qi, blood, Yin or Yang and poor nutrition of heart in patients with congenital constitutional insufficiency, chronic disease or loss of blood; by attack of heart by phlegm and fire pathogen due to deficiency of heart qi, exhaustion of Yin and blood or stagnation of heart qi; or by stagnation of qi and blood and blockage of heart and blood vessels due to invasion of heat pathogen into heart. The severe patients may have collapse and crisis due to deficiency of heart Yang.

(2) Differential diagnosis

1) Qi deficiency type: The patients may suffer from incontrollable palpitation of heart, frightening, mental tiredness, shortness of breath, spontaneous sweating, difficulty to fall asleep, white thin tongue coating and thready pulse.

2) Blood deficiency type: The patients may suffer from palpitation of heart aggravated by worriment and tiredness, sallow complexion, dizziness, vertigo, poor memmory, insomnia, pink tongue proper and thready rapid pulse.

3) Phlegm fire type: The patients may suffer from intermittent palpitation of heart induced by frightening, chest distress, agitation, insomnia, dreaminess, repeated interruption of sleep, dryness and bitter taste in mouth, spitting of much sticky sputum, discharge of dark urine, constipation, yellow greasy tongue coating and stringy slippery pulse.

4) Blood stasis type: The patients may suffer from persistent and gradually aggravated palpitation of heart, chest distress, shortness of breath after physical exertion, paroxysmal pricking pain in heart and chest, cyanotic lips and tongue and uneven, knotted or intermittent pulse. The chronic patients with deficiency of heart Yang may suffer from continuous palpitation of heart, cold body and limbs, orthopnea, edema and almost impalpable feeble pulse.

(3) Treatment

The reducing technique of eye acupuncture is applied at heart acupoint in 6th region to patients with excessive syndrome and the needles are retained for a longer time; and the reinforcing technique is applied at the same acupoint with moxibustion for a longer time to treat the patients with deficient syndrome. The middle energizer acupoint in 5th region is added to tonify heart qi, settle fright and calm mind for patients with qi deficiency; the spleen acupoint in 7th region is added to tonify heart and calm mind for patients with blood deficiency; the lung acupoint in 1st region and stomach acupoint in 7th region are added to resolve phlegm, clear heat, settle fright and calm mind for patients with phlegm fire; and the liver acupoint in 4th region is added to promote circulation of qi and blood, release blood stasis and strengthen heart for patients with blood stasis. The eye acupuncture is applied once a day and the needles are retained for 15 − 20 min.

(4) Clinical experience

The eye acupuncture can produce an apparent effect to treat palpitation of heart due to various causes and improve cardiac function. The therapeutic effect is closely related to the selection of acupoints and application of technique. The stimulation of acupuncture applied for palpitation of heart must be very gentle. A combined therapy is applied to the patients of coronary heart disease, angina pectoris and other organic diseases of heart according to the differential diagnosis of syndrome. The therapeutic effect of acupuncture for tachycardia is better than that for bradycardia and it is poor for myocardiopathy.

16. Xiongbi (chest pain)

The Xiongbi is a disease in traditional Chinese medicine with pain and distress in chest radiated to back and accompanied with colic pain in chest, shortness of breath and asthma in severe cases.

(1) Etiology and pathogenesis

The Xiongbi may be caused by invasion of cold pathogen to block flow of Yang in chest of patients with Yang deficiency in the past; by accumulation of endogenous phlegm and dampness pathogen; or by failure to disperse Yang and stagnation of qi and blood in chest of people always working at the desk without enough physical exercise over a long period of time.

(2) Differential diagnosis

The patients with a mild Xiongbi may suffer from chest distress and unsmooth breath; the severe cases may suffer from chest pain radiated to back, shortness of breath, asthma and even sudden onset of chest pain, pale complexion, extremely cold limbs, sweating and feeble pulse; the patients of deficient cold type may suffer from chest pain exacerbated by attack of coldness, chillness and cold limbs; the patients of turbid phlegm type may suffer from cough to spit much sputum; and the patients of blood stasis type may suffer from pricking pain in chest and dark purple lips and tongue.

(3) Treatment: To promote flow of Yang and expel pathogen.

The even reinforcing and reducing technique of eye acupuncture is applied at heart acupoint in 6th region and the needle is retained for 5 – 15 min, once a day in 5 days as a therapeutic course and a rest for 2 days is arranged between 2 courses. The moxibustion and cupping therapy may be applied at Danzhong (CV 17, at the midpoint between 2 nipples) acupoint and back Shu acupoints for patients of deficient cold and turbid phlegm types.

(4) Clinical experience

The symptoms of Xiongbi may be found in many diseases of western medicine and they should be accurately diagnosed and independently treated with their effective medicines and therapies if the eye acupuncture can not produce any effect. Otherwise, the patients may miss an opportunity of cure because of a delay. The patients should be on a dietary regime with more vegetables and less oily food and take an easy life.

17. Angina pectoris

The angina pectoris is a syndrome caused by a sudden ischemia and hypoxia of myocardium.

The patients may suffer from a sudden onset of pain behind the upper and middle segments of sternum and on the left side of anterior midline and the pain may be radiated to the shoulder, neck, back and upper limb, usually to the left shoulder and left arm. The pain is colic, pricking or cutting in nature and an attack of pain may last for 3 - 5 min and occasionally over 10 min. At the same time, they also show pale complexion, frightening, cold sweating and dyspnea. The heart rhythm is irregular and the premature beats often occur. A systolic murmur over the apex of heart and a rough systolic murmur over the aortic valve region can be heard. The hypertrophy of heart and hypertension are often found.

The atypical pain of angina pectoris may occur in precordial region, upper limb, neck, throat or back and sometimes the patients may also have some symptoms of digestive system.

The ECG may be normal during the remission period, but some abnormal changes can be found during the attack of this disease, such as depressed ST segment, lowered T wave and even hypertrophy of left ventricle and bundle - branch block in chronic patients.

Treatment: To expand chest and adjust qi and blood.

The upper energizer acupoint in 3rd region and heart acupoint in 6th region are selected to do eye acupuncture and Danzhong (CV 17) and Neiguan (PC 6, 2 cun proximal to the carpal crease and between ulna and radius bones) acupoints are selected to do body acupuncture. The effective medicines should be administered for critical patients.

18. Edema

The edema is a symptom occurring in many diseases with body fluid accumulated in skin, muscles, head, face, orbit, limbs, abdomen and even whole body.

(1) Etiology and pathogenesis

The impairment of the function of lung to disperse qi may cause blockage of water channel to transport water to urinary bladder and the accumulated water may combine with the wind pathogen in body surface to produce edema; the attack of dampness pathogen to spleen may disturb the function of spleen to transport body fluid and the water may be accumulated in body and spread to skin and muscles to cause edema; in patients with pyogenic sores the toxic pathogen of sores may attack lung and spleen to interfere their functions to disperse qi and transport body fluid and to cause edema;

the transporting and distributing the functions of lung and spleen may be imperilled by the inadequate diet to cause accumulation of water and edema; the damage of spleen and kidney by overfatigue and indulgence of sexual activity may disturb the transporting function of spleen Yang to cause edema; and the patients with deficiency of kidney may lose the function of evaporating and discharging water to develop edema.

(2) Differential diagnosis

1) Yang type of edema: The patients may suffer from edema spread from head to whole body, more remarkable in upper body and pitting in nature with a quick refilling of the pit, shiny skin, reduction of urine, chillness, fever, soreness and pain of body, cough and rough breath. The patients of edema caused by wind-cold pathogen may have cold body, no sweating, white slippery tongue coating and floating tense pulse; and the patients of edema caused by wind-heat pathogen may have sore throat, yellow thin tongue coating and floating rapid pulse.

2) Yin type of edema: The patients with deficiency of spleen may suffer from edema spread from feet to whole body, more remarkable in lower body and pitting in nature with a slow refilling of the pit, dull skin, re-

duction of urine, fullness of upper abdomen, diarrhea with loose stool, tiredness of limbs, white greasy tongue coating and soft moderate pulse; and the patients with deficiency of kidney may suffer from pain and soreness of waist and leg, cold limbs, mental tiredness, white thin tongue coating and deep, thready and weak pulse.

(3) Treatment

1) Yang type of edema: The reducing technique of eye acupuncture is applied at lung acupoint in 1st region and spleen and stomach acupoints in 7th region to expel wind pathogen, disperse lung qi, discharge water and resolve edema.

2) Yin type of edema: The even reinforcing and reducing technique is applied at kidney acupoint in 2nd region and spleen and stomach acupoints in 7th region to strengthen spleen, warm kidney, enrich Yang and discharge water. The technique to produce more reducing effect is applied to patients with strong constitution and the reinforcing technique is applied to patients with apparent deficiency of spleen and kidney.

(4) Clinical experience

In patients of acute and chronic nephritis at early or middle stage the body acupuncture at Shangxing

(GV 23), Sibai (ST 2), Jiache (ST 6), Renzhong (GV 26), Chengjiang (CV 24), Shousanli (LI 10), Pianli (LI 6), Baxie (EX-UE 9), Fulin (KI 7), Zulinqi (GB 41) and Xianqu (ST 43) acupoints may be applied with eye acupuncture. In patients of chronic nephritis with deficiency of lung, spleen and kidney the moxibustion may be applied with moxa cone changed for 5 − 7 times, twice a day. The critical patients with oliguria or auria, distension of abdomen, palpitation of heart, cyanotic face and lips, nausea, vomiting, foul smell from mouth, bleeding of nose and teeth, coma, delirium, convulsion of limbs and deep breath should be rescued by a combined therapy.

The patients should pay attention to arrange a healthy life and prevent common cold. The sea food is prohibited and the intake of salt should be limited.

The Yang type of edema is easy to cure, but it may develop into Yin type of edema if not adequately treated and nursed; and the Yin type of edema can be controlled in most patients by a prolonged acupuncture treatment and proper nursing care.

19. Headache

The headache is a common subjective symptom occurring in many diseases and it can be divided into headache due to attack of external pathogens and damage of internal organs according the etiology of headache; or classified into Taiyang, Shaoyang, Yangming and Jueyin types according to the location of pain.

(1) Etiology and pathogenesis

The headache in most patients is caused by attack of external wind pathogen, because it is the most active one among 6 external pathogens. The wind may combine with cold, heat or dampness pathogen to attack the head and eyes and block circulation of qi and blood; the emotional disturbance and mental depression may cause transformation of stagnated qi into fire pathogen to attack head and eyes; and the headache of liver Yang type is caused by the attack of Yang wind pathogen to head in patients with deficiency of kidney water and excessive liver wind.

The headache of blood deficiency type is caused by deficiency of qi and blood and poor supply of blood to head in patients with weak spleen and stomach, chronic diseases or loss of blood; the headache of turbid phlegm type is due to overeating of sweet and greasy food which may produce turbid phlegm to attack the brain in obese people; and the headache may also be caused by stagnation of blood and blockage of meridians due to external trauma.

(2) Differential diagnosis

1) External pathogen type: The onset of a severe headache caused by external pathogen is prompt and it is often accompanied with other symptoms caused by external pathogens. The patients may suffer from headache with tense sensation in head aggravated by blowing wind, chillness, fever and running nose with clear nasal discharge caused by wind-cold pathogen; suffer from distending headache, flushed face, thirst and running nose with yellow nasal discharge caused by wind-heat pathogen; or they may suffer from headache with heaviness, tiredness without desire to move their body and limbs, poor appetite and diarrhea caused by wind dampness pathogen.

2) Liver Yang type: The patients may suffer from a spastic pain on both sides of head induced by emotional disturbance, fury, yellow thin tongue coating and

stringy pulse; and the deficiency of kidney water may cause tinnitus, deafness, soreness of waist and emission of semen.

3) Blood deficiency type: The patients may suffer from a lingering headache with a dull and empty sensation, tiredness, cold limbs, palpitation of heart, sallow complexion, pale tongue proper with thin coating and thready pulse.

4) Turbid phlegm type: The patients may suffer from an aching and heavy sensation in head as wrapped by a piece of cloth, distress in upper abdomen, vomiting of sputum and saliva, white greasy tongue coating and slippery pulse.

5) Blood stasis type: The patients with a history of external trauma may suffer from a repeated attack of pricking pain at fixed region of head, purple tongue proper with ecchymoses and uneven pulse.

In addition, the headache can also be classified according to the location of pain. The pain of Taiyang headache is on occipital region and radiated to nape and back; the pain of Yangming headache is on forehead and superciliary ridge; the pain of Shaoyang headache is on temporal and ear region; and the pain of Jueyin headache is on the vertex of head and radiated to Muxi (tie of eye).

(3) Treatment

The upper energizer acupoint in 3rd region and other acupoints of eye selected according to differential diagnosis of syndrome are used to apply eye acupuncture.

The lung acupoint in 1st region is used for headache of external pathogen type to expel wind pathogen; the liver acupoint in 4th region is used for headache of liver Yang type to calm liver and subdue Yang; the spleen and stomach acupoints in 7th region, liver acupoint in 4th region and kidney acupoint in 2nd region are used for headache of blood deficiency type to tonify spleen and stomach and adjust qi and blood; the spleen and stomach acupoints in 7th region and lung acupoint in 1st region are used for headache of turbid phlegm type to strengthen spleen and stomach and resolve phlegm and dampness; and liver acupoint in 4th region and spleen acupoint in 7th region are used for headache of blood stasis type to release blockage of meridian and adjust collateral.

The acupoints may also be selected according to the inspection of blood vessels and the location of headache if the patients do not suffer from other apparent general symptoms.

Besides upper energizer acupoint in 3rd region, the following acupoints can be selected acording to the location of headache. The urinary bladder acupoint in 2nd region and small intestine acupoint in 6th region are selected for Taiyang headache in occipital region; the stomach acupoint in 7th region and large intestine acupoint in 1st region are selected for Yangming headache in frontal region; the gallbladder acupoint in 4th region is selected for Shaoyang headache in temporal region; and the liver acupoint in 4th region is selected for Jueyin headache in parietal region. The acupoints are selected to promote circulation of qi and blood through their related meridians.

The reducing technique is used for headache caused by external pathogens; and the reinforcing or even reinforcing and reducing technique is used for headache caused by injury of internal organs according to the differential diagnosis of pure excessive or deficient syndrome or a mixed syndrome of deficiency and excessiveness. The body acupuncture can be used in combination with eye acupuncture. The needle should be inserted backward at Taiyang (EX-HN 5) acupoint for temporal headache and other needles are horizontally inserted beneath scalp.

(4) Clinical experience

The eye acupuncture can produce an apparent effect to relieve headache, but the patients with severe headache should be carefully examined to correctly evaluate the causes of headache and make a correct diagnosis of the primary disease for not misdiagnosing and mismanaging the serious diseases with headache as an early symptom.

20. Facial palsy

This is a disease with paralysis of facial muscles and it is a Zhongluo (attack of collateral) syndrome of Zhongfeng (stroke) disease. It is also called Kouyan Waixie (deviation of mouth and eye) in traditional Chinese medicine.

(1) Etiology and pathogenesis

The facial palsy is due to the deficiency of qi and blood, invasion of wind and cold pathogens to meridians and muscles on face and blockage of meridian; or due to transformation of hyperactive liver Yang into wind pathogen and the attack of this endogenous wind pathogen to Yangming and Taiyang meridians to cause spasm of muscles and blood vessels, abnormal circulation of qi and blood and paralysis of muscles on diseased side of face.

(2) Differential diagnosis

1) Attack of wind and cold pathogen: The onset of this disease is prompt and in the morning as brushing teeth the patients may suddenly find the paralysis of facial muscles on one side, disappearance of frontal wrinkles, increase of eye fissure, flat nasolabial groove, deviation of drooped mouth angle to the normal side more remarkable as showing teeth and smiling, failure to frown and raise eyebrow, close eye, blow up cheek and protrude lips together with shedding tears, slurred speech, slobbering and retention of food debris between teeth and cheek. Some patients may have pain behind ear and impairment of taste sensation at anterior 2/3 of tongue. The tongue coating is white and thin and the pulse is tense.

2) Ascent of hyperactive liver Yang: Refer to the discussion in apoplexy (stroke).

(3) Treatment

In the early stage, the reducing technique of eye acupuncture is first applied at upper energizer acupoint in 3rd region and then at liver and gallbladder acupoints in 4th region by horizontal insertion of No. 32 needles of 1.5 cm in length, once a day for 10 times as a therapeutic course. The lung acupoint in 1st region may be added for facial palsy caused by attack of wind and cold pathogens; the spleen and stomach acupoints in 7th region may be added for patients with deficiency of vital energy; the body acupuncture may be applied at Zusanli (ST 36) acupoint to produce a needling sensation travelling upward through knee to abdomen for chronic patients over 3 months.

(4) Clinical experience

The early treatment with eye acupuncture can produce a good effect for facial palsy. The patients should protect themselves from further attack of wind and cold pathogens. Some sequelae may be retained in chronic patients over 6 months and the moxibustion with ginger can produce certain effect to treat the sequelae of facial palsy.

21. **Apoplexy (stroke)**

The patients of this disease may suddenly develop hemiplegia, deviation of mouth, stiffness of tongue, slurred speech and coma and it can be divided into types of attack to meridians and attack to internal organs.

(1) Etiology and pathogenesis

This is a disease in patients over middle age and its basic pathogenesis is the gradual exhaustion of essence, deficiency of liver and kidney Yin and hyperactivity of liver Yang. The stroke may be caused by stagnation of heart and liver qi to produce fire pathogen and phlegm due to emotional disturbance and mental depression; or by production of heat pathogen from phlegm accumulated in obese patients due to indulgence of alcohol and overeating of greasy, spicy and fried food. The sudden attack of stroke is often induced by violent emotional disturbance and careless living.

The stroke due to attack to meridians at superficial part of body is caused by adverse invasion of liver wind with phlegm to meridians to produce blood stasis and the patients may only suffer from mild symptoms, including numbness of limbs, hemiplegia, deviation of mouth and slurred speech.

The stroke due to attack to internal organs can be divided into excessive (closed) pattern and deficient (open) pattern. The excessive pattern is caused by sudden rushing up of wind and Yang together with phlegm and fire pathogen; by disturbed circulation of qi and blood to attack brain; and by disturbance of Yin and Yang and blockage of orifices of heart by phlegm and heat pathogen and the patients may suddenly fall down and lose consciousness. The deficient pattern is caused by excessive phlegm and fire pathogen derived from liver Yang, failure to conquer pathogens due to deficiency of vital energy (body resistance) as well as dissociation and exhaustion of Yin and Yang.

(2) Differential diagnosis

1) Attack to meridian type: The symptoms are less severe and the patients are mentally clear. They may suffer from numbness and sluggish movement of limbs on one side, deviation of mouth and eye, slobbering from mouth angle, slurred speech, yellow thin or greasy tongue coating and stringy slippery pulse.

2) Attack to internal organ type: The symptoms are acute and severe and the patients may suddenly fall down and lose consciousness. They may also suffer from hemiplegia, deviation of mouth, slobbering from mouth angle, stiffness of tongue and aphonia. This type of stroke can be further divided into excessive (closed) and deficient (open) patterns. The patients of excessive pattern may suffer from mental confusion, locked jaw, flushed face, rough breath, clenching of

fists, contraction of body, sputum wheezing in throat, constipation, retention of urine, red tongue proper with yellow coating and slippery rapid or stringy tense pulse; and the patients of deficient pattern may suffer from coma, pale complexion, open mouth and closed eyes, shallow breath, limp hands and cold limbs, incontinence of urine and stool and deep, thready, feeble and weak pulse.

(3) Treatment

1) Attack to meridian type: The No. 32 needles of 1.5 cm in length are horizontally inserted 6 mm from the orbital edge at upper energizer acupoint in 3rd region and middle energizer acupoint in 5th region while the eyelid is tightened by a finger of the physician and the needle are retained for 5 – 15 min, once a day for 12 times as a therapeutic course. The involved limbs are actively or passively moved or massaged in the period with needles retained.

2) Attack to internal organ type: The oblique or horizontal insertion of No. 32 needles of 1.5 cm in length is applied at upper energizer acupoint in 3rd region, lower energizer acupoint in 8th region and liver and gallbladder acupoints in 4th region for patients of excessive pattern and at upper energizer acupoint in 3rd

region, lower energizer acupoint in 8th region and spleen and stomach acupoints in 7th region for patients of deficient pattern and the needles are retained for 15 min, once a day.

(4) Clinical experience

The eye acupuncture can produce an apparent effect to treat the sequelae of stroke. The manipulation of acupuncture must be very gentle in the acute stage of stroke and especially in patients with cerebral hemorrhage or increased blood pressure or intracranial pressure. The acupuncture may be postponed until the stabilization of disease in critical patients, but it should be started as early as possible after the disease is stable for obtaining a better therapeutic result to recover the locomotive function of limbs. In general, an apparent effect can be obtained in the early 3 months. A combined therapy should be adopted to rescue the critical patients and to treat the chronic patients with muscular atrophy and disuse of limbs. The warm moxibustion can be used to treat patients with deficiency of qi and blood. The patients should be on a dietary regime with low fat and high protein and they should maintain a calm mood.

Appendix: Hemiplegia after brain trauma.

The flaccid paralysis of limbs on one side of body

and incontinence of urine after brain trauma or brain operation can be treated with eye acupuncture at bilateral upper energizer acupoints in 1st region, lower energizer acupoints in 8th region and kidney acupoint in 2nd region with the needles retained for 20 min, once a day for 10 times as a therapeutic course. A combined therapy with acupuncture should be started from the early recovery period of the disease.

22. Insomnia

The patients with insomnia may have difficulty to fall asleep, wakening from time to time or sleeplessness through whole night.

(1) Etiology and pathogenesis

The insomnia may be caused by injury of heart and spleen by worriment and mental tiredness and deficiency of qi and blood to nourish the mind; by wasting of kidney Yin due to sexual intemperance, hyperactivity of heart fire and loss of interaction between heart and kidney; by damage of spleen and stomach by excessive intake of food, production of phlegm from excessive dampness pathogen, transformation of accumulated phlegm to heat pathogen and attack of phlegm and heat pathogen to mind; or by injury of liver by mental depression and anger and transformation of stagnated liver qi to fire pathogen to attack the mind.

(2) Differential diagnosis

1) Deficiency of heart and spleen: The patients may suffer from insomnia, dreaminess, easy wakening, palpitation of heart, poor memory, tiredness, sallow complexion, poor appetite, diarrhea, pale tongue proper with white thin coating and thready weak pulse.

2) Deficiency of Yin and excessiveness of fire pathogen: The patients may suffer from insomnia, vexation, easy wakening, hot sensation in heart, palms and soles, frightening, sweating, dryness in mouth and throat, dizziness, tinnitus, poor memmory, soreness of waist, emission of semen, irregular menstruation, red tongue proper and thready rapid pulse.

3) Internal disturbance of phlegm and heat pathogen: The patients may suffer from unsteady sleep, annoyance, distress in chest and upper abdomen, spitting of profuse sputum, dizziness, vertigo, bitter taste in mouth, yellow greasy tongue coating and slippery or stringy pulse.

4) Upward flaming of liver fire pathogen: The patients may suffer from dizziness, headache, vexation,

anger, difficulty to fall asleep, red eyes, tinnitus, pain in flanks, bitter taste in mouth, yellow thin tongue coating and stringy rapid pulse.

(3) Treatment

The reinforcing or even reinforcing and reducing technique is used to apply eye acupuncture at upper energizer acupoint in 3rd region, kidney acupoint in 2nd region and heart acupoint in 6th region for insomnia of all types, once a day in the afternoon or at night before going to bed for calming the mind. The middle energizer acupoint in 5th region and spleen and stomach acupoints in 7th region may be added to tonify heart and spleen for insomnia due to deficiency of heart and spleen; the kidney acupoint in 2nd region and liver acupoint in 4th region may be added to tonify Yin and reduce fire pathogen for insomnia due to deficiency of Yin and excessiveness of fire pathogen; the stomach and spleen acupoints in 7th region are added to release blood stasis and clear heat for insomnia due to internal disturbance of fire pathogen; and the liver and gallbladder acupoints in 4th region are added to suppress liver and reduce fire pathogen for insomnia due to upward flaming of liver fire pathogen.

(4) Clinical experience

As a common symptom, the insomnia may produce much trouble to the work and learning of patients. The acupuncture can produce a good effect to treat insomnia without any side effect and it is more effective as performed in afternoon or at night. The psychological factor is also important in the pathogenesis of insomnia, the psychotherapy is therefore a useful treatment to patients with insomnia too.

23. Vertigo

The vertigo is a subjective symptom with blurred vision, nausea, vomiting, and rotating sensation in brain as sitting in a boat or car.

The vertigo may be caused by ascent of hyperactive liver Yang produced by emotional disturbance and attack of stirred Yang wind pathogen to the head and eyes; by impairment of digestive function of spleen due to overeating of sweet and greasy food in obese people and formation of phlegm from dampness pathogen to cloud the clear mind; by deficiency of heart and spleen due to extreme worriment in weak people and deficiency of qi and blood to nourish the head and eyes; or by deficiency of kidney essence and emptiness of brain.

(2) Differential diagnosis

1) Ascent of active liver Yang: The patients may suffer from dizziness, vertigo, headache, aggravation of symptoms by tiredness and anger, high irritability, anger, flushing face, bitter taste in mouth, red tongue proper with white thin coating and stringy pulse.

2) Blockage by turbid phlegm: The patients may suffer from heaviness of head as wrapped by a piece of cloth, blurred vision, distress in chest and upper abdomen, vomiting of sputum and saliva, no appetite, white greasy tongue coating and slippery or soft pulse.

3) Deficiency of qi and blood: The patients may suffer from lingering dizziness, blurred vision, mental tiredness, sallow complexion, palpitation of heart, insomnia, aggravation of symptoms after tiredness, pale tongue proper and thready pulse.

4) Deficiency of kidney essence: The patients may suffer from persistent vertigo, blurred vision, mental tiredness, intolerance to tiredness, soreness and weakness of waist and knees, emission of semen, irregular menstruation, red tongue proper and deep thready pulse.

(3) Treatment

The upper energizer acupoint in 3rd region is used

for vertigo of all types. The liver acupoint in 4th region is added to suppress liver Yang for vertigo due to ascent of hyperactive liver Yang; the stomach acupoint in 7th region is added to adjust stomach and resolve phlegm for vertigo due to blockage of turbid phlegm; the middle energizer acupoint in 5th region is added to tonify qi and blood for vertigo due to deficiency of qi and blood; and the kidney acupoint in 2nd region is added to tonify kidney essence for vertigo due to deficiency of kidney essence. The reducing technique is used to treat vertigo due to ascent of hyperactive liver Yang or blockage of turbid phlegm and the reinforcing technique is used to treat vertigo caused by deficiency of qi and blood or deficiency of kidney essence. The eye acupuncture with needles retained may be applied once a day or twice a day during the episode of vertigo.

(4) Clinical experience

The eye acupuncture may produce an apparent effect to control the acute attack of vertigo in patients with hypertension, anemia, neurasthenia or auditory vertigo, but it is ineffective in patients with vertigo due to damage of auditory nerve by some antibiotics.

24. Emission of semen

The emission of semen is a symptom in adult men with semen spontaneously discharged with or without dream of sexual activity during sleep and it is a normal phenomenon with emission of semen once a week in adult without other symptoms. The emission of semen in patients of neurasthenia, prostatitis and seminal vesiculitis in western medicine can be treated by the following methods.

(1) Etiology and pathogenesis

The emission of semen with dream is due to deficiency of heart and kidney Yin and excessiveness of monarch and ministerial fire or due to irritation to seminal vesicle by the damp-heat pathogen produced from improper diet and accumulated in lower energizer; and the emission of semen without dream is due to exhaustion of primordial qi of kidney and insecurity of semen gate and the severe emission without dream is due to deficiency of heart and kidney.

(2) Differential diagnosis

1) Emission with dream: The patients may suffer

from spontaneous discharge of semen with dream, no impotence, unsteady sleep, premature ejaculation of semen, red tongue proper and thready rapid pulse. The dizziness, tinnitus, soreness in waist, discharge of dark urine may occur in chronic patients.

2) Emission without dream: The patients may suffer from spontaneous discharge of semen induced by any sexual desire, impotence, pale complexion, soreness and coldness in waist and knees, mental and physical tiredness, spontaneous sweating, shortness of breath, pale tongue proper with white coating and thready or thready rapid pulse.

(3) Treatment

The lower energizer acupoint in 8th region is used to do eye acupuncture for both types of emission; and Guanyuan (CV 4) acupoint is used to do body acupuncture.

1) Emission with dream: The heart acupoint in 6th region, kidney acupoint in 2nd region and spleen acupoint in 7th region may be used to clear heart fire and communicate heart and kidney.

2) Emission without dream: The kidney and urinary bladder acupoints in 2nd region are used to tonify kidney qi and secure semen gate.

The emission of semen can be divided into excessive and deficient types and the emission with dream is the excessive type with a short clinical course and low frequency of emission. The patients are asked to empty their urinary bladder for downward inserting needle at Guanyuan (CV 4) acupoint to produce a needling sensation to the perineum. The emission without dream is a deficient type with symptoms of kidney deficiency through a long clinical course and it may be treated with moxibustion or reinforcing technique of acupuncture at Guanyuan (CV 4) acupoint.

(4) Clinical experience

The eye acupuncture can produce an apparent effect to treat emission of semen, but a long therapeutic course of treatment is necessary for chronic patients of emission without dream. The psychotherapeutists can help the patients to arrange a regular and healthy life and abolish the worriment about their disease. In patients with emission refractory to all treatments should have a thorough examination to rule out important organic lesions in reproductive system. They should also perform physical exercise to improve their health. An eye acupuncture at urinary bladder acupoint in 2nd region alone can be applied to treat emission caused by accumulation of damp-heat pathogen in lower energizer.

25. Impotence

The impotence is usually caused by exhaustion of kidney essence and deficiency of fire in Mingmen (life gate) due to indulgence of sexual activity; caused by damage of heart and kidney by extreme worriment or frightening; or occasionally caused by downward pouring of damp-heat pathogen.

The patients of deficient type may suffer from poor erection of penis, spontaneous discharge of thin and cold semen, dizziness, tinnitus, pale complexion, mental tiredness, shallow breath, soreness and weakness of waist and knees, hatred of coldness, cold limbs, pale tongue proper and thready weak pulse; and the patients of excessive type may suffer from poor erection of penis or erection without enough firmness for sexual intercourse, premature ejaculation of semen, wet scrotum with bad smell, soreness and heaviness of lower limbs, discharge of dark urine, yellow greasy tongue coating and soft rapid pulse.

Treatment: The lower energizer acupoint in 8th region is used for eye acupuncture and Dahe (KI 12) acupoint for body acupuncture. The reinforcing technique of eye acupuncture is applied to tonify kidney Yang for deficient type of impotence; and the even reinforcing and reducing technique is used to clear damp-heat for excessive type of impotence. The kidney acupoint in 2nd region is also used for deficient type; and the kidney acupoint in 2nd region and spleen acupoint in 7th region are also selected for excessive type of impotence.

26. Stiff neck

This is a disease of locomotive system with pain, rigidity and limitation of movement of neck. The muscular sprain and muscular rheumatism of neck, occipital neuralgia and hyperplasia of cervical spine in western medicine can be treated by the following methods.

(1) Etiology and pathogenesis

This disease may be caused by spasm of neck muscles after stretch or sprain of muscles for a long time at night as sleeping in an improper posture or with an inadequate pillow; by acute sprain or chronic strain; or by attack of external wind-cold pathogen to produce blockage of meridians and stagnation of qi and blood.

(2) Clinical manifestations

After getting up in the morning, the patients may suddenly feel stiffness and pain on one side of neck, radiated to the shoulder, back and upper arm of the same side. They may also suffer from headache and chillness, if the disease is caused by the attack of wind-cold pathogen. The local muscular spasm and tenderness can be relieved by hotness.

(3) Treatment: To adjust qi and blood and release blockage of meridians.

A No. 32 needle of 1.5 cm in length is clockwise and horizontally inserted at upper energizer acupoint in 3rd region of left eye and the needle is counterclockwise inserted on right eye. The reducing or even reinforcing and reducing technique is applied and the needles are retained for 15 - 20 min, once a day. The patients are asked to move their neck during the treatment. The local moxibustion and cupping therapy can adjust qi and blood and release blockage of meridians.

(4) Clinical experience

The eye acupuncture can produce a good effect to treat the stiff neck and the muscular spasm can be relieved after 2 - 3 times of treatment. If the stiff neck repeatedly relapses in patients above 40 years of age, they may suffer from cervical spondylosis and the traction with massage may produce a better therapeutic effect on them.

27. Trigeminal neuralgia

This is a disease with paroxysmal attacks of burning pain in the distributing area of trigeminal nerve and it is called Mian Tong (facial pain) or Meilenggu Tong (pain of eyebrow bone) in wind syndrome of traditional Chinese medicine.

(1) Etiology and pathogenesis

This disease is caused by the attack of external wind-cold pathogen to block the circulation of qi and blood in meridians; caused by stagnation of liver qi and transformation of liver qi to fire pathogen; or caused by adverse ascent of fire pathogen from stomach.

(2) Differential diagnosis

1) Wind-cold type: The patients may suffer from paroxysmal attacks of pricking or burning pain on face, slight chillness, white thin tongue coating and floating or floating rapid pulse.

2) Deficient fire type: The patients may suffer from paroxysmal attacks of spastic pain induced by

brushing teeth or chewing food, local hot sensation, annoyance, anger and yellow thin tongue coating.

(3) Treatment

The eye acupuncture is applied at upper energizer acupoint in 3rd region and spleen and stomach acupoints in 7th region to expel wind-cold pathogen and promote circulation of qi in meridians for wind-cold type and the needles are retained for 20 min; and the eye acupuncture is applied at upper energizer acupoint in 3rd region and liver and gallbladder acupoints in 4th region to clear liver fire for deficient fire type and the needles are retained for 5 - 15 min. The reducing technique is applied for excessive syndrome at early stage and the even reinforcing and reducing technique is applied for chronic patients of wind-cold type. The moxibustion may be applied at the acupoints on face.

(4) Clinical experience

The eye acupuncture can produce an apparent effect to treat this disease. If the effect is not apparent after eye acupuncture is appliedfor 1 - 2 therapeutic courses, the patients should be carefully examined to find other causes of facial pain.

28. Intercostal neuralgia

This is a disease with paroxysmal exacerbation of pain in costal region and it is called Xie Tong (pain in flank) or Xiong Tong (pain in chest) in traditional Chinese medicine.

(1) Etiology and pathogenesis

This disease is caused by stagnation of liver qi in meridians due to mental depression or fury; or caused by blood stasis in meridians due to external trauma.

(2) Differential diagnosis

1) Qi stagnation type: The patients may suffer from wandering pain over chest, chest distress, belching, induction of symptoms by emotional disturbance, anger, insomnia, white thin tongue coating and strong stringy pulse.

2) Blood stasis type: The patients with history of chronic chest pain or external trauma may suffer from persistent pain fixed in location and distension in flanks worse at night, hatred of palpation on chest, occasional appearance of petechiae or ecchymoses on tongue and stringy or thready uneven pulse.

(3) Treatment

The eye acupuncture is applied at middle energizer acupoint in 5th region and liver acupoint in 4th region to disperse liver qi and stop pain for qi stagnation type; and it is applied at middle energizer acupoint in 5th region, liver acupoint in 4th region and spleen acupoint in 7th region to promote circulation of qi and blood and relieve pain for blood stasis type. Because the excessive syndrome is more common in this disease the reducing technique is usually used; but in chronic patients the reinforcing technique is used after application of reducing technique first. The reducing technique is applied to treat blood stasis type with needles not retained.

(4) Clinical experience

The effect of eye acupuncture is apparent to treat this disease and it is better to treat the idiopathic intercostal neuralgia. The primary disease of secondary costal neuralgia must be adequately treated to eliminate the basic etiological factor.

29. Neuralgia sciatica

This is a disease with pain distributed along the pathway and innervating area of sciatic nerve and it is called Yaotui Tong (pain of waist and leg) in traditional Chinese medicine.

(1) Etiology and pathogenesis

This disease is caused by invasion of cold and dampness pathogens to produce disturbance of Ying (nutritive material) and Wei (defensive energy) and blockage of circulation of qi through meridians in patients with deficiency of liver and kidney and deficiency of qi and blood in meridians; caused by invasion of cold and dampness pathogens to block meridians and collaterals after living in damp environment, drench with rain or sitting on wet ground for a long time; or caused by stagnation of qi and blood to block meridians after sprain, contusion or collision to body or carrying very heavy burden on body.

(2) Differential diagnosis

1) Kidney deficiency type: The patients may suffer from pain and weakness of waist and leg exacerbated after tiredness and reduced after rest, sallow complexion, listlessness, difficult walking, pale, red or crimson tongue proper with white thin coating and deep, thready and soft pulse.

2) Cold dampness type: After invasion of external pathogens, the patients may suffer from a sudden onset

of pain within a limited segment of the nerve or radiated to either direction of it and accompanied with numbness, white thin or white greasy tongue coating and deep uneven or tense pulse; and the patients attacked by damp-heat pathogen derived from damp-cold pathogen may suffer from burning pain along the nerve, constipation, yellow greasy tongue coating and rapid uneven pulse.

3) External trauma type: The patients with history of external trauma may suffer from radiating pain from waist through hip region to leg unrelievable by changing posture, limitation of movement, red tongue proper with yellow thin coating and uneven tense pulse.

(3) Treatment

The No. 32 needles of 1.5 cm in length are used to apply eye acupuncture by vertical or horizontal insertion underneath skin for 1 cm at lower energizer acupoint in 8th region and kidney acupoint in 2nd region without twisting, lifting and thrusting stimulation and they are retained for 5 – 15 min.

The reducing technique of eye acupuncture or acupuncture plus moxibustion is applied for cold dampness type; the reducing technique may also be applied for damp-heat and external trauma types; the reinforcing technique of eye acupuncture with moxibustion is applied for kidney deficiency type; and the even reinforcing and reducing technique is applied for chronic patients. The cupping therapy may be applied at acupoints with apparent tenderness.

(4) Clinical experience

The eye acupuncture can produce an apparent effect to treat neuralgia sciatica. The therapeutic effect is better in cold dampness type than in external trauma and deficient types; and it is better in trunk type than in root type.

30. Lumbago

The lumbago is a common symptom of many diseases with pain in the spinal column or on its one or both side, The lumbago in diseases of spinal column, acute sprain of waist and chronic muscular strain in western medicine can be treated by the following methods.

(1) Etiology and pathogenesis

The lumbago may be caused by invasion of cold and dampness pathogens to block circulation of qi and blood in meridians after catching cold, sitting on wet ground or drench with rain; by disturbance of qi and blood due to standing and sitting in an improper posture for a long time or due to damage of meridians and collaterals by external trauma to produce stagnation of qi and blood; or by deficiency of kidney, exhaustion of essence and blood and poor nourishment of meridians in aged people, chronic patients or people with intemperance of sexual activity.

The lumbago is closely related to kidney, because the waist is a house of kidney and the kidney is connected with spinal column and many meridians.

(2) Differential diagnosis

1) Cold dampness type: The patients may suffer from pain, coldness, soreness, numbness and heaviness in waist radiated to sacral, hip, thigh and popliteal regions after the attack of wind, cold and dampness and the sufferings can be exacerbated by the change of weather, coldness and raining.

2) Qi and blood stagnation type: The patients with history of chronic injury and strain of waist may suffer from fixed pain and spasm of muscles in waist with limitation of movement; and the patients with history of acute injury or sprain of waist may suffer from severe lumbago and limitation of movement.

3) Kidney deficiency type: The patients may suffer from a dull pain, soreness, weakness and emptiness in waist with a gradual onset and a chronic course, aggravation of pain after tiredness and alleviation of pain after lying in bed. The patients with deficiency of kidney Yang may suffer from mental tiredness, cold limbs, emission of semen, weakness of knees and deep thready pulse; and the patients with deficiency of kidney Yin may suffer from annoyance, insomnia, flushing face and thready rapid pulse.

(3) Treatment

The lower energizer acupoint in 8th region may be used to apply eye acupuncture for lumbago of all types. The liver and gallbladder acupoints in 4th region are added to treat acute lumbago; and the upper energizer acupoint in 3rd region and kidney acupoint in 2nd region are added to treat chronic lumbago. The needles are retained for 20-30 min and the patients are asked to move their waist during the treatment. The reducing or even reinforcing and reducing technique is used to treat lumbago of cold dampness type or qi and blood stagnation type; and the reinforcing technique is used to treat the kidney deficiency type. The bleeding therapy applied at Weizhong (BL 40) acupoint is used to treat sprain of waist.

(4) Clinical experience

The therapeutic course for acute sprain of waist is short and 1 or 2 therapeutic course of eye acupuncture is enough to cure the lumbago; the therapeutic course must be long enough to treat lumbago of cold dampness and kidney deficiency types. The persistent acupuncture and cupping therapy can at least temporarily control or relieve the lumbago due to diseases of spinal columm.

31. Periarthritis of shoulder (frozen shoulder)

This is a disease of soft tissue injury in shoulder with pain and limitation of movement and it is common in people around 50 years old. It is a disease included in Bi-syndrome in traditional Chinese medicine.

(1) Etiology and pathogenesis

This disease is caused by external trauma, chronic strain or attack of external pathogens to produce stagnation of qi and blood in meridians, poor nutrition of muscles and blood vessels, atrophy and adhesion of muscles and functional disturbance of shoulder joint.

(2) Clinical manifestation

At the early stage, the patients may suffer from pricking pain around shoulder and radiated to neck and elbow, worse at night to interfere sleep, fright at the attack of wind and coldness to shoulder, tenderness in a big area around shoulder and limitation of movement of shoulder joint; and the chronic patients may suffer from severe functional disturbance and muscular atrophy, but the pain may be reduced.

(3) Treatment

The upper energizer acupoint in 3rd region and liver and gallbladder acupoints in 4th region are used for this disease of all types. The upper energizer acupoint in 3rd region is selected for patients with pain in triple energizer meridian aggravated by forward extension of arm; the small intestine acupoint in 6th region is selected for patients with pain in small intestine meridian aggravated by backward extension of arm; and the region with abnormal blood vessels on eye (usually the liver and gallbladder acupoints in 4th region) is selected for patients with pain in 3 hand Yang meridians aggravated by abduction of arm. The needles are vertically inserted for $0.7 - 1$ cm or obliquely in a $15° - 30°$ angle for 1.5 cm and they are retained for 10 min and the handle of needle is scratched once in each interval of 5 min. The treatment is applied once a day for 10 times as a therapeutic course and a rest of 3 days is arranged between 2 courses.

(4) Clinical experience

The eye acupuncture can produce an apparent effect on relieving pain and improving movement at the early stage of frozen shoulder, but it is useless in chronic patients with adhesion of shoulder joint. The combination of massage and this treatment can reduce the sufferings and improve the locomotive function of shoulder joint. The patients should perform physical exercise and keep the local warm.

32. Wei-syndrome (paralysis)

This is a disease with weakness of limbs (usually lower limbs) and atrophy of muscles. The multiple neuritis, myelitis, progressive myatrophy, myasthenia gravis and paralegia with muscular paralysis in western medicine can be treated with the following methods.

(1) Etiology and pathogenesis

The Wei-syndrome is caused by the attack of heat pathogen to lung, wasting of body fluid and poor nourishment of muscles and blood vessels; by the flaccidness of muscles and immobility of joints due to attack of external dampness pathogen after living in wet environment or drench with rain; by deficiency of essence and blood and poor nutrition of blood vessels, muscles and bones due to injury of kidney in weak patients with chronic diseases or in people with intemperance of sexual activity; by retention of lochia to attack the waist and legs in women after delivery of baby; or by blood stasis and poor nourishment of meridians and blood vessels due to external trauma.

(2) Differential diagnosis

1) Wasting of body fluid by heat pathogen in lung: During or after the febrile infectious disease, the patients may suffer from fever, preference for coolness, annoyance, thirst, discharge of dark urine in short stream, constipation, red tongue proper with yellow coating and thready rapid pulse.

2) Steaming of damp-heat pathogen: The patients may suffer from distress in chest and upper abdomen, tiredness of limbs, slight edema, greasy tongue coating and soft rapid pulse.

3) Deficiency of liver and kidney: The chronic patients may suffer from weakness of waist and knees,

vertigo, red tongue proper with scanty coating and thready rapid pulse.

4) Blood stasis: The patients with a history of childbirth or external trauma may suffer from numbness of limbs, reduction or loss of sensation, purple lips and tongue proper and uneven pulse.

(3) Treatment

The upper energizer acupoint in 3rd region is used to do eye acupuncture for paralysis of upper limb; the lower energizer acupoint in 8th region and kidney acupoint in 2nd region are used for paralysis of lower limbs; and the lower energizer acupoint in 8th region and gallbladder acupoint in 4th region is used for heel pain.

The reinforcing technique is used for paralysis due to deficiency of liver and kidney and the reducing technique is used for other types. The plum-blossom acupuncture may be applied for blood stasis.

(4) Clinical experience

The Wei-syndrome in traditional Chinese medicine contains many organic and functional diseases of western medicine, therefore, the correct diagnosis should be made before treatment for obtaining an ideal therapeutic effect. In chronic patients a combined treatment with medicines and physical therapy may improve the therapeutic result. The early treatment of acupuncture can prevent and postpone the progress of muscular atrophy.

33. Bi-syndrome (arthritis)

The Bi-syndrome is a disease of traditional Chinese medicine due to blockage of circulation of qi and blood in muscles, blood vessels and joints with soreness, pain, numbness, heaviness, swelling and immobility of joints caused by invasion of external pathogens.

(1) Etiology and pathogenesis

The Bi-syndrome is caused by invasion of wind, cold and dampness pathogens in patients with deficiency of qi, blood, Yin and Wei. The dominance of 3 pathogens is diffenent in different patients, the dominance of wind pathogen may cause wandering Bi-syndrome and the dominance of dampness pathogen may cause fixed Bi-syndrome. In patients with excessive Yang qi and accumulation of heat pathogen in body the heat Bi-syndrome is easily produced.

(2) Differential diagnosis

1) Wandering Bi-syndrome: The patients may suffer from wandering pain in joints and muscles, limita-

tion of movement, white thin tongue coating and floating or floating rapid pulse and some patients may have low fever and chillness.

2) Aching Bi-syndrome: The patients may suffer from severe pain at fixed location with aggravation by coldness and alleviation by hotness, limitation to flex and extend joints, white, thin and greasy tongue coating and stringy tense pulse.

3) Fixed Bi-syndrome: The patients may suffer from aching pain at fixed location in joints and muscles with exacerbation in raining day, heaviness, numbness, white, thick and greasy tongue coating and soft thready or thready uneven pulse.

4) Heat Bi-syndrome: The patients may suffer from arthralgia with local redness, swelling, hotness and tenderness, limitation of movement, thirst, fever unrelievable by sweating, yellow greasy tongue coating and slippery rapid or large full pulse.

(3) Treatment

The lower energizer acupoint in 8th region is used to do eye acupuncture and Dubi (ST 35) acupoint is used to do body acupuncture for Bi-syndrome of all types. The reducing technique is applied at liver acupoint in 4th region to expel wind pathogen and relieve pain for wandering Bi-syndrome; the reducing technique is applied at stomach acupoint in 7th region to expel cold pathogen and stop pain for aching Bi-syndrome; the even reinforcing and reducing technique is applied at spleen acupoint in 7th region to strengthen spleen and eliminate dampness pathogen for fixed Bi-syndrome; and the reducing technique is applied at large intestine acupoint in 1st region to clear heat pathogen for heat Bi-syndrome, 1–2 times a day at acute stage and once every 2 days at chronic stage for 10 times in total as a therapeutic course.

(4) Clinical experience

The Bi-syndrome in traditional Chinese medicine is correspondent to rheumatic arthritis, tenosynovitis, peripheral neuritis and rheumatoid arthritis in western medicine. The acupuncture can produce an apparent analgesic effect, but it can not cure those diseases. The heat Bi-syndrome and the fixed Bi-syndrome with a normal antistreptolysin-O test are particularly difficult to treat.

The patients should enrich the intake of nutrients and take an easy life and at the same time they should avoid eating irritative food and protect themselves from the attack of wind, cold and dampness pathogens.

34. Sprain of soft tissues

In traditional Chinese medicine it is called Shangjin (injury of soft tissues) with local swelling and pain and impairment of movement caused by acute injury of soft tissues in trunk and limbs.

(1) Etiology and pathogenesis

The soft tissues may be injured by severe contusion, sprain, falling down or collision during violent physical exercise or caused by carrying heavy burden to produce injury of meridians and blood vessels, stagnation of qi and blood and blockage of circulation of qi in meridians.

(2) Clinical manifestations

The patients may suffer from local bruise, swelling, pain, tenderness, functional disturbance of joints and limitation of movement.

(3) Treatment

The upper energizer acupoint in 3rd region is used for injury of neck, chest and upper limb; the middle energizer acupoint in 5th region is selected for injury of chest and back; and the lower energizer acupoint in 8th region is chosen for injury of waist and lower limb. Other acupoints may also selected according to the inspection of blood vessels on eye. The patients take a sitting or lying flat posture and the needles are horizontally or obliquely inserted and gently twisted in a frequency of 150 times per min for 1 – 2 min. After the needling sensation is obtained the needles are retained for 10 – 30 min and they are again twisted after each 5 – 10 min interval. The eye acupuncture is applied once a day.

(4) Clinical experience

The eye acupuncture can produce an apparent effect on treating acute sprain of waist after 1 – 2 times of treatment. The patients are asked to move their waist during the treatment. The cupping therapy and moxibustion can be applied for patients with marked local swelling 24 hours after the injury.

35. Irregular menstruation

This is a common gynaecological disease with abnormal change of menstrual cycle and amount, color and nature of menstrual discharge.

(1) Etiology and pathogenesis

The irregular menstruation is due to overeating of cold and uncooked food or invasion of external cold pathogen to cause blood stasis and blockage of meridians; due to formation of endogenous fire pathogen from stagnated liver qi to cause disturbanceof blood circulation and disharmony of Chongmai (thoroughfare vessel) and Renmai (conceptional vessel); due to worriment or improper diet to cause damage of spleen, deficiency of spleen and stomach qi and disturbance of blood circulation; due to exhaustion of Yin and blood in patient with chronic disease or loss of blood; due to deficiency of kidney qi and failure to adjust filling and drainage of Xuehai (blood reservoir); or due to mental depression, stagnation of liver qi, blockage of Chongmai and Renmai and impediment of blood circulation.

(2) Differential diagnosis

1) Cold syndrome: The patients may suffer from delayed menstrual cycle to discharge a small amount of pink menstrual blood with blood clots, pain in lower abdomen relievable by hotness, hatred of coldness, cold limbs, white thin tongue coating and slow pulse.

2) Heat syndrome: The patients may suffer from antedated menstrual cycle to discharge profuse, dark purplish red and sticky menstrual blood, annoyance,

thirst, flushing face, red eyes, anger, pain and distension in flanks, red tongue proper with yellow coating and stringy rapid pulse.

3) Deficient syndrome: The menstrual cycle may be either antedated or postponed and the menstrual discharge is less in amount, pale in color and thin in nature. The patients may also suffer from poor appetite, mental tiredness and diarrhea, if their spleen and stomach are deficient; they may suffer from palpitation of heart, dizziness, blurred vision and sallow complexion, if their heart and spleen are deficient; and they may suffer from vertigo, tinnitus, soreness of waist, pain and empty sensation in lower abdomen, pale tongue proper and thready pulse, if the liver and kidney are deficient.

4) Excessive syndrome: The menstrual cycle may be antedated or delayed and the menstrual discharge is less in amount, purplish black in color and mixed with blood clots. The patients may suffer from mental depression, pain in flanks, pain and distension in lower abdomen, purple tongue proper and stringy uneven pulse.

(3) Treatment

The eye acupuncture is applied at lower energizer

acupoint in 8th region, liver acupoint in 4th region and kidney acupoint in 2nd region for this disease. The reinforcing technique is applied for deficient syndrome; the reducing technique is applied for excessive syndrome; and the moxibustion is applied to abdomen for cold syndrome.

(4) Clinical experience

The eye acupuncture can produce an ideal effect to treat this disease. It should be started 5 – 7 days before the menstrual period and continued to the beginning of menstruation.

36. Dysmenorrhea

This is a disease of women with pain (or severe pain) in lower abodomen before, during or after menstrual period.

(1) Etiology and pathogenesis

The dysmenorrhea may be caused by mental depression, stagnation of liver qi, blockage of blood circulation in Chongmai and Renmai and accumulation of blood in uterus; by invasion of cold and dampness pathogens into uterus to produce coagulation of blood due to drench with rain, walking across cold water in river, intake of cold food and drink or sitting or lying on wet ground; by deficiency of qi and blood in weak people or chronic patients, emptiness of Xuehai (blood reservoir) and poor supply of nutrition to blood vessels of uterus; by impediment of uterine discharge due to deficiency of Yang qi and impairment of blood circulation; or by damage of liver and kidney and exhaustion of essence and blood to nourish blood vessels of uterus in people with intemperance of sexual activity or in multiparous women to produce dysmenorrhea after menstrual period.

(2) Differential diagnosis

1) Stagnation of qi and blood: The menstrual blood is small in amount, discharged by drops and mixed with purple blood clots. The patients may suffer from distension of chest, flanks and breasts, purple tongue proper with petechiae and deep stringy pulse.

2) Stagnation of cold and dampness pathogens: The patients may suffer from coldness, pain and tenderness in lower abdomen before or during menstruation radiated to lumbar region and relievable by hotness, white thin tongue coating and deep tense pulse. The menstrual discharge is less in amount, dark red in color

and mixed with blood clots.

3) Deficiency of qi and blood: The menstrual discharge is pale and thin and the patients may suffer from dull pain in lower abdomen during or after menstrual period and relievable by pressing lower abdomen, sallow complexion, pale tongue proper with thin coating and thready weak pulse. The patients with deficiency of Yang may have chillness and diarrhea; and the patients with deficiency of liver and kidney may have dizziness, tinnitus and aching in lumbar region.

(3) Treatment

The lower energizer aucpoint is used to do eye acupuncture for dysmenorrhea of all types. The liver and gallbladder acupoints in 4th region and spleen acupoint in 7th region are used to disperse liver qi, promote blood circulation and release blood stasis for stagnation of qi and blood type of dysmenorrhea; the spleen acupoint in 7th region and middle energizer acupoint in 5th region are used to eliminate cold and dampness pathogens, release stagnation in meridians and control pain for stagnation of cold and dampness pathogens; and the stomach and spleen acupoints in 7th region and middle energizer acupoint in 5th region are used to tonify qi and blood and adjust Chongmai and Renmai for deficiency of qi and blood.

The eye acupuncture is applied 5 − 7 days before the menstrual period once a day and the needles are retained for 20 min. The reducing technique is applied for excessive syndrome; and the reinforcing technique is applied for deficient syndrome with the moxibustion applied on the lower abdomen. The eye acupuncture should be continued for 2 − 3 months.

(4) Clinical experience

Besides controlling pain the eye acupuncture can also improve the general condition and endocrinal function of human body, adjust menstrual cycle and enhance the function of reproductive organs in pelvis. The acupuncture should be started 5 − 7 days before the menstrual period and the treatment should be applied for 2 − 4 cycles of menstruation. If the eye acupuncture can not produce an apparent effect to stop dysmenorrhea, the patients should receive a thorough gynaecological examination to rule out any important organic lesions. They should avoid overfatigue, mental strain, attack of cold weather and intake of cold and uncooked food.

37. Hyperemesis gravidarum

This is a common disease at early stage of pregnancy with nausea, vomiting, anorexia, food preference or regurgitation right after intake of food.

(1) Etiology and pathogenesis

This disease is caused by stoppage of menstruation after pregnancy, overflow of excessive qi in Chongmai (thoroughfare vessel) and Renmai (conceptional vessel) to attack stomach and loss of adjusting and descending function of stomach; by poor transporting function of deficient spleen, accumulation of endogenous phlegm and dampness pathogen in upper abdomen and upward rushing of qi in Chongmai with phlegm and dampness pathogen; by deficiency of liver blood and excessiveness of liver qi after the supply of most Yin and blood in body to nourish fetus; or by damage of liver by mental depression and fury, loss of dispersing function of liver and upward rushing of qi in Chongmai with liver qi to attack stomach to produce nausea and vomiting.

(2) Differential diagnosis

1) Deficiency and weakness of spleen and stom-

ach: At early stage of pregnancy the women may suffer from nausea, vomiting, anorexia, regurgitation right after intake of food, spitting of clear saliva, mental tiredness, sleepiness, pale tongue proper with white coating and moderate, slippery and weak pulse. The patients with accumulation of turbid phlegm may suffer from fullness in chest and upper abdomen, vomiting of sputum and saliva and white greasy coating.

2) Disharmony between liver and stomach: At early stage of pregnancy, the women may suffer from regurgitation of sour fluid, fullness of chest, pain in flanks, belching, sighing, mental depression, distension of head, dizziness, thirst, bitter taste in mouth, yellow thin tongue coating and stringy slippery pulse.

(3) Treatment

The middle energizer acupoint in 5th region and spleen and stomach acupoints in 7th region are used to apply eye acupuncture for deficiency and weakness of spleen and stomach; and the middle energizer acupoint in 5th region and liver and gallbladder acupoints in 4th region are used for disharmony between liver and stomach. The reducing technique is used for excessive syndrome; and the reinforcing technique is used for deficient syndrome and the needles are retained for 15 min, once a day.

(4) Clinical experience

The therapeutic effect of eye acupuncture for this disease is apparently good. At early stage of pregnancy the acupuncture should be applied with less needles and gentle stimulation. In patients with mild symptoms, the sufferings can be relieved after 3 − 4 times of treatment; and in severe cases, the symptoms can be reduced after 2 − 3 times of treatment. The administration of medicines is not necessary, but the infusion of fluid is indicated in patients with apparent dehydration due to repeated vomiting. The patients should keep a calm mood, take enough rest in bed and follow a dietary regime of small frequent meals and they should avoid eating cold, greasy and uncooked food.

38. Oligogalactia (reduction of milk secretion)

This is a symptom of women after childbirth with reduced secretion of milk not enough to feed their babies.

(1) Etiology and pathogenesis

The oligogalactia is due to deficiency of nutrient

sources to produce milk after loss of too much blood during labor or in women with a weak and lean body in the past; or caused by emotional disturbance and stagnation of liver qi to block the ducts of breasts.

(2) Differential diagnosis

1) Deficiency of qi and blood: The milk is small in amount and thin in nature and the breasts are not painful and distended. The patients may also suffer from dizziness, palpitation of heart, sallow complexion, poor appetite, tiredness and weakness, pale tongue proper with scanty coating and feeble thready pulse.

2) Stagnation of qi and blockage of milk ducts: The patients may suffer from pain and distension of breasts radiated to flanks without any secretion of milk, chest distress, distension of upper abdomen, mental depression, thin tongue coating and stringy pulse.

(3) Treatment

The reinforcing technique of eye acupuncture is applied at spleen and stomach acupoints in 7th region and heart and small intestine acupoints in 6th region for deficiency of qi and blood type of this disease; and the reducing technique is applied at stomach acupoint in 7th region, small intestine acupoint in 6th region and liver acupoint in 4th region for stagnation of qi and blockage of milk ducts.

(4) Clinical experience

The eye acupuncture can produce a better therapeutic effect to treat the oligogalactia due to stagnation of qi and blockage of milk ducts; and the rich nutrient supply is also very important in the treatment of oligogalactia due to deficiency of qi and blood.

39. Incontinence of urine (bed wetting)

This is a disease of children above 3 years of age with urine spontaneously discharge during sleep at night.

(1) Etiology and pathogenesis

The kidney is a partner organ of urinary bladder with an exterointerior relationship between them and it can play a role in the control of discharge of urine and stool. The deficiency of kidney qi may impair the function of urinary bladder to control the discharge of urine. The lung are the upper source of water and the spleen can distribute body fluid. Therefore, the incontinence of urine may occur if the spleen and lung qi is deficient and the discharge of urine is disturbed. The accumulation of damp-heat pathogen in lower energizer and the transformation of this pathogen into fire may attack urinary bladder to cause incontinence of urine.

(2) Differential diagnosis

1) Deficiency of kidney qi: The patients may have repeated bed wetting at night, soreness of waist, weakness of legs, mental tiredness, general weakness, pale complexion, cool limbs, poor intelligence, discharge of clear urine in long stream, pale tongue proper and thready pulse.

2) Deficiency of spleen and lung qi: The patients may suffer from bed wetting during sleep, shallow breath, no desire to speak, leanness of body, mental tiredness, sallow complexion, poor appetite, diarrhea, spontaneous sweating, red tongue proper with white thin coating and thready weak pulse.

3) Damp-heat pathogen in lower energizer: The patients may suffer from urgent discharge of small amount of yellow foul urine, high irritability, talking and gritting teeth in sleep, dryness in mouth, red lips, yellow tongue coating and thready rapid pulse.

(3) Treatment

The eye acupuncture is applied at lower energizer acupoint in 8th region and kidney acupoint in 2nd region to tonify primordial qi of kidney and secure normal discharge of urine for deficiency of kidney type of bed wetting; the acupuncture at lower energizer acupoint in 8th region, spleen and stomach acupoints in 7th region and lung acupoint in 1st region is applied to tonify spleen qi and secure normal urination for deficiency of spleen and lung qi; and the acupuncture at lower energizer acupoint in 8th region, urinary bladder acupoint in 2nd region and liver acupoint in 4th region is applied to clear liver heat and release blockage in water channel for accumulation of damp-heat pathogen in lower energizer. The even reinforcing and reducing technique is used for damp-heat type; and the reinforcing technique is used for other deficient types.

(4) Clinical experience

The physicians and nurses must be very kind to manage the children and abolish their fright and sadness. The children should avoid mental excitement and drinking much water before going to bed. The X-ray film of lumbar and sacral spinal vertebrae should be taken to rule out congenital occult cleft spine if the eye acupuncture does not produce any effect.

40. Urticaria

The urticaria is a skin disease with pink or white itching papules coming and going quickly from time to time. The acute patients at early stage may be easily cured after a short period of treatment; but the chronic urticaria may relapse repeatedly for several months.

(1) Etiology and pathogenesis

The urticaria may be caused by the attack of bad weather and invasion and accumulation of wind pathogen in skin and muscles; by intake of sea food or accumulation of parasites in body; or by heat pathogen accumulated in stomach and intestine and transferred to and accumulated in skin and muscles to produce urticaria.

(2) Differential diagnosis

The skin rashes often suddenly appear as fresh red, pink or white papules unevenly distributed over the skin with severe itching and they may quickly disappear as the prompt change of blowing wind.

1) Invasion of wind pathogen: The patients may also suffer from chillness, fever, cough, aching in

limbs, white thin tongue coating and floating rapid pulse besides the skin rashes.

2) Accumulation of heat pathogen in stomach and intestine: The patients may also suffer from pain in abdomen, mental tiredness, poor appetite, constipation or diarrhea, yellow greasy tongue coating and slippery rapid pulse.

(3) Treatment

The eye acupuncture may be applied at lung and large intestine acupoints in 1st region and spleen acupoint in 7th region to disperse wind pathogen and adjust Ying (nutritive material) and Wei (defensive energy) qi for invasion of wind pathogen type; and the acupuncture at lung and large intestine acupoints in 1st region and stomach acupoint in 7th region to clear heat in Yangming meridians and adjust qi and Ying for accumulation of heat pathogen in stomach and intestine. The reducing or even reinforcing and reducing technique is used to treat this disease, because it is an excessive syndrome. The eye acupuncture is applied once a day or twice a day for patients with severe itching.

(4) Clinical experience

The eye acupuncture can produce certain effect to relieve itching and promote subsidence of skin rashes and it is especially useful in acute urticaria, but the remote effect is not good. Therefore, after the resolution of skin rashes, the eye acupuncture treatment should be continued for a longer period of time to prevent the relapse. A combined therapy can be used to treat the chronic patients refractory to many therapies or patients who have been treated with large dosage of cortisone. At the same time, the etiological and inducing factors should be found and eliminated for prevention of relapses.

41. Eczema

This is a common skin disease with symmetrical skin lesions and paroxysmal severe itching.

(1) Etiology and pathogenesis

The eczema is caused by invasion of wind, dampness and heat pathogens to block circulation of qi and blood or by poor nutrition of skin and muscles due to deficiency of blood and production of endogenous wind and dryness pathogens from heat pathogen in body.

(2) Differential diagnosis

1) Damp-heat type: At the early stage, the local skin becomes itching and fresh red in color and the ery-

thema, papules and some ulcers may appear in succession. After scratching, the skin lesions become erosive in appearance to exude yellow fluid and to form crusts, but no permanent scars are retained after the crusts are peeled off. The patients may also suffer from abdominal pain, constipation or diarrhea, discharge of dark urine in short stream, fever, headache, thin or yellow greasy tongue coating and floating rapid or slippery rapid pulse.

2) Blood deficiency type: This is a chronic skin disease derived from acute eczema with a long clinical course and repeated relapses. The skin lesions are dark in color, rough, thickened and in a lichenous appearance with a clear margin. The tongue proper is pale with white thin coating and the pulse is thready and stringy.

(3) Treatment

The lung and large intestine acupoints in 1st region and spleen and stomach acupoints in 7th region are used to do eye acupuncture to clear damp-heat pathogen, adjust collaterals and stop itching for eczema of damp-heat type; and the eye acupuncture at spleen and stomach acupoints in 7th region and lung acupoint in 1st region is applied to tonify blood, moisten dryness, clear heat in blood and relieve itching for eczema of blood deficiency type.

The reducing technique is used to treat acute eczema, because it is usually caused by damp-heat pathogen; and the reinforcing technique is used to treat chronic eczema, because it is due to deficiency of blood and the moxibustion may be applied over the chronic lesion until the local skin becomes flushed. For severe itching the plum-blossom acupuncture may be applied over the lesion until the local skin is flushed with slight oozing of blood.

(4) Clinical experience

This is a stubborn skin disease with repeated relapses. The eye acupuncture may produce an apparent effect to relieve itching and the bleeding cupping therapy can produce certain effect to treat chronic eczema. The sea food and irritative food are prohibited to eat.

42. Furuncle and carbuncle

The furuncle and carbuncle are the common surgical diseases and they may occur at any part of human body, usually on the face, hand and foot. At the early stage, the lesion of furuncle is small, firm and with a deep root as a nail, it is therefore called Dingchuang (nail sore) in traditional Chinese medicine.

(1) Etiology and pathogensis

The furuncle and carbuncle are caused by accumulation of toxic heat pathogen in internal organ in patients with intemperance of alcohol and greasy and spicy food; by poor hygiene of skin, external trauma, infection of skin and accumulation of qi and blood in meridians; or by invasion of excessive toxic heat pathogen into internal organs to produce a critical disease.

(2) Clinical manifestation

At the begining, a small vesicle like a grain of millet appears on the skin with a deep root as a nail and with local itching, numbness, redness, swelling, pain and burning sensation. Following the spread of local infection, the patients may suffer from severe local pain, chillness, fever and thirst; and the further rapid progress of local infection may cause high fever, restlessness, vomiting, coma and delirium and it is called Dingchuang Zouhuang (Carbuncle with septicemia).

(3) Treatment

The reducing technique of eye acupuncture is applied at acupoints selected according to inspection of blood vessels on eye. The moxibustion with moxa cones can be applied after the application of eye acupuncture and the body acupuncture can be applied around the lesions.

(4) Clinical experience

The skin lesions should not be pressed or squeezed and the alcohol, smoking and spicy and sea food are prohibited. The eye acupuncture can be used to treat the furuncle at early stage and the patients should be transferred to surgical department for surgical treatment if the eye acupuncture can not produce any therapeutic effect.

43. Hemorrhoids

The hemorrhoids inside the dentate line of anus are the internal hemorrhoids; the hemorrhoids outside the dentate line are the external hemorrhoid; and those scattered on both sides of dentate line are the mixed hemorrhoids. The patients may suffer from local pain and swelling and passage of bloody stool during the acute attack of hemorrhoids.

(1) Etiology and pathogenesis

The hemorrhoids may be caused by intake of spicy, greasy, fried, cold and uncooked food, working in a persistent sitting or standing posture, habitual constipation, multiple delivery of babies or chronic dysentery to produce disturbance of qi and blood, blockage of meridians and downward pouring of turbid qi and stagnated blood to anus.

(2) Clinical manifestation

The patients of internal hemorrhoids may suffer from passage of bloody stool without pain except after infection; and the patients of external hemorrhoids may suffer from severe pain and a sensation of foreign body in anus without discharge of blood in stool.

(3) Treatment:

The reducing technique of eye acupuncture is applied at the eye acupoints selected according to inspection of blood vessels on eyes for the hemorrhoids due to accumulation of damp-heat pathogen; and the reinforcing technique is applied for hemorrhoids due to descending of deficient qi and the moxibustion is applied at Baihui (GV 20) acupoint, once a day during the acute attack and once every 2 days during the remission period.

(4) Clinical experience

The eye acupuncture can produce an apparent effect to stop bleeding, relieve pain and reduce the size of hemorrhoids and it may be used in combination with operation and administration of medicines to treat the large hemorrhoids, mixed hemorrhoids and anal fistula. The patients should establish a good habit of regular bowel movement and the spicy food is prohibited.

44. Ptosis of eyelid

This is a symptom with upper eyelid drooped down to overlap the pupil and disturb the vision and it can be divided into the congenital and acquired types. In general, the eyelid of only one eye is involved in the latter type. The eye type of myasthenia gravis and paralysis of oculomotor nerve with ptosis of eyelid in western medicine may be treated by the following methods.

(1) Etiology and pathogenesis

The ptosis of eyelid may be caused by congenital deficiency of kidney qi; by functional disturbance of muscles and blood vessels due to attack of external wind pathogen; by deficiency of spleen qi and flaccidness of muscles; or by injury of muscles and blood vessels by external trauma.

(2) Differential diagnosis

The important symptoms of this disease are drooping down of upper eyelid to overlap pupil and interfere vision, paralysis of external ocular muscles, poor rotation of eyeball and double vision.

1) Deficiency of spleen qi: The patients may suffer from mental tiredness, poor appetite, vertigo, sallow complexion, paralysis of eyelid and feeble and weak pulse. 2) Invasion of external wind pathogen: The onset of ptosis of eyelid is prompt with paralysis of other muscles.

(3) Treatment

The spleen acupoint in 7th region and upper energizer acupoint in 3rd region are used to do eye acupuncture for ptosis of eyelid of all types. The reinforcing technique is applied at stomach acupoint in 7th region to tonify qi and release blockage of collaterals for ptosis of eyelid due to deficiency of spleen and stomach qi; and the reducing technique is applied at gallbladder acupoint in 4th region and large intestine acupoint in 1st region to expel wind pathogen and release blockage of collaterals for this disease due to invasion of external wind pathogen.

(4) Clinical experience

The eye acupuncture can produce an apparent effect to treat ptosis of eyelid in patients with paralysis of oculomotor nerve, myasthenia gravis and external trauma, but it is not effective to treat congenital ptosis of eyelid.

45. Strabismus (wall-eye)

This is an eye disease with inability of both eyes to simultaneously look straight forward. The paralytic strabismus and concomitant strabismus in western medicine can be treated by the following methods.

(1) Etiology and pathogenesis

The wall-eye may be caused by deficiency of spleen and stomach qi, emptiness of collaterals and invasion of wind pathogen or by deficiency of essence and blood of liver and kidney to nourish Muxi (tie of eye).

(2) Differential diagnosis

The important symptoms of this disease are deviation of pupil to medial or lateral side in one or both eye, impediment of rotation of eyeball and double vision.

1) Invasion of wind pathogen: The onset is prompt and the patients may also suffer from headache, fever, nausea, vomiting, white tongue coating and

floating pulse.

2) Deficiency of liver and kidney: The onset is insidious and the patients may suffer from dizziness, vertigo, blurred vision, tinnitus, pale tongue proper and deep thready pulse.

(3) Treatment

To expel wind pathogen, release blockage of collaterals and adjust eye muscles.

The large intestine acupoint in 1st region, small intestine acupoint in 6th region, urinary bladder acupoint in 2nd region, stomach acupoint in 7th region and upper energizer acupoint in 3rd region are used to do eye acupuncture to treat this disease of all types. The liver acupoint in 4th region and kidney acupoint in 2nd region are added to treat strabismus due to deficiency of liver and kidney. The body acupuncture may be applied with the eye acupuncture. For medial strabismus Taiyang (EX-HN 5), Sizhukong (TE 23) and Tongziliao (GB 1) acupoints are used; and for lateral strabismus Cuanzhu (BL 2) and Jingming (BL 1) are used.

(4) Clinical experience

The eye acupuncture can produce a better effect on treating traumatic paralysis of external eye muscles, but it is less effective in chronic patients with strabismus caused by acute infectious diseases. The piercing acupuncture is applied at body acupoints around the eye and the skin must be carefully sterilized for eye acupuncture into orbit to prevent infection. The needle holes should be pressed for a while to prevent bleeding after removal of needles.

46. **Hordeolum (stye)**

This is an eye disease with a small, itching and painful induration on the border of eyelid and it is called Zhenyan (pin of eye):

(1) Etiology and pathogenesis

The stye is caused by the attack of wind-heat pathogen to the eyelid to produce stagnation of qi and blood or by improper intake of food to produce accumulation of heat pathogen in spleen and stomach and upward ascent of heat pathogen to attack the eye.

(2) Differential diagnosis

At the beginning of disease, the patients may feel itching and pain on the border of eyelid and on which a small red induration appears. The local pain is gradually exacerbated and particularly worsened while lowering the head. The lesion may spontaneously resolve in patients with a small induration; but the severe lesion may form a small abscess and it may heal after rupture and complete drainage of pus.

1) Invasion of wind-heat pathogen: The patients may also suffer from chillness, fever, headache, thin tongue coating and floating pulse.

2) Accumulation of heat pathogen in spleen and stomach: The patients may have foul smell from mouth, dryness in month, annoyance, yellow greasy tongue coating and rapid pulse.

(3) Treatment

The eye acupuncture is applied at upper energizer acupoint in 3rd region and liver acupoint in 4th region to expel wind and clear heat pathogen for invasion of wind-heat pathogen type; and the acupuncture at upper energizer acupoint and spleen acupoint in 7th region is applied to clear toxic-heat pathogen for accumulation of heat pathogen in spleen and stomach type. The reducing technique is applied for both types and the eye acupuncture is applied once a day.

(4) Clinical experience

At the early stage, the acupuncture can promote

the absorption and resolution of inflammation and swelling and relieve the pain; and after formation of abscess, it can promote the suppuration and drainage of pus. The therapeutic effect of eye acupuncture is better before the suppuration of lesion.

47. Red eye (conjunctivitis)

This is an acute symptom occurring in many eye diseases with redness, swelling and pain of eyes. They are usually the infectious eye diseases, such as acute conjunctivitis and epidemic keroconjunctivitis, common in spring and autumn seasons.

(1) Etiology and pathogenesis

The red eye is caused by invasion of toxic wind-heat pathogen to block the circulation of meridianal qi or by the upward invasion of excessive fire pathogen in liver and gallbladder to produce accumulation of qi and blood and blockage of meridians.

(2) Differential diagnosis

1) Invasion of toxic wind-heat pathogen: The patients may suffer from redness, swelling, pain and dryness of eyes difficult to open, photophobia, lachrymation, headache, fever and floating rapid pulse.

2) Excessive fire pathogen in liver and gallbladder: The patients may suffer from redness, swelling and pain of eyes, photophobia, lachrymation, bitter taste in mouth, annoyance, hot sensation in body and stringy pulse.

(3) Treatment

The eye acupuncture is applied at large intestine acupoint in 1st region and gallbladder acupoint in 4th region to clear wind-heat pathogen, resolve swelling and stop pain for invasion of toxic wind-heat pathogen type; and the acupuncture is applied at liver and gallbladder acupoints in 4th region and upper energizer acupoint in 3rd region to clear fire pathogen in liver and gallbladder for the excessive fire pathogen from liver and gallbladder type. The bleeding therapy may be applied at Taiyang (EX-HN 5) acupoint.

(4) Clinical experience

The eye acupuncture is a simple and effective method to treat acute conjunctivitis. The needles are horizontally and counterclockwise inserted underneath skin to apply the reducing technique at all eye acupoints and the needles are retained for 15 min, once a day.

48. Induction of lachrymation by wind

This is a symptom occurring in many eye diseases, such as keratitis and iridocyclitis with stimulation of trigeminal nerve, facial nerve or pterygopalatine nerve. The spontaneous lachrymation in those diseases of western medicine can be treated with the following methods.

(1) Etiology and pathogenesis

The spontaneous lachrymation may be caused by attack of wind pathogen in patients with exhaustion of essence and blood and deficiency of liver and kidney or by attack of wind pathogen in patients with excessive liver fire pathogen.

(2) Differential diagnosis

1) Deficiency of liver and kidney: The patients may suffer from spontaneous lachrymation of clear tears induced by blowing wind, blurred vision at late stage, dryness in eyes, no redness and pain in eyes, red tongue proper and thready stringy pulse.

2) Excessiveness of liver fire: the patients may suffer from redness, swelling and pain of eyes, photo-

phobia, lachrymation of sticky turbid tears induced by wind, yellow thin tongue coating and stringy rapid pulse.

(3) Treatment

The reinforcing technique of eye acupuncture is applied at liver and gallbladder acupoints in 4th region and kidney acupoint in 2nd region to tonify liver and kidney for deficiency of liver and kidney type; and the reducing technique is applied at large intestine acupoint in 1st region and liver and gallbladder acupoints to expel wind and clear heat pathogen, disperse liver qi and improve vision for excessiveness of liver fire type.

(4) Clinical experience

The therapeutic effect of acupuncture is better in patients of this disease caused by excessiveness of liver fire than that by deficiency of liver and kidney or than in aged peoplewith spontaneous lachrymation at winter time.

49. **Qingmang (optic nerve atrophy)**

This is a disease of eye with gradual impairment of vision but the appearance of outer eye is normal. The progressive blindness of optic nerve atrophy in western medicine can be treated by the following methods.

(1) Etiology and pathogenesis

The optic nerve atrophy with impaired vision is caused by deficiency of essence, blood and Yin of liver, kidney and heart.

(2) Differential diagnosis

The visual field is gradually decreased and the visual acuity is reduced to complete blindness and the patients often suffer from headache.

1) Deficiency of liver and kidney Yin: The patients may suffer from dryness in eyes, dizziness, tinnitus, soreness of waist, emission of semen, red tongue proper and thready pulse.

2) Deficiency of heart Yin: The patients may suffer from vertigo, annoyance, palpitation of heart, poor memmory, unsteady sleep, red tongue proper and feeble weak pulse.

(3) Treatment

The reinforcing technique of eye acupuncture at upper energizer acupoint in 3rd region and nearby acupoints including Chengqi (ST 1) and Qiuhou (EX-HN 7) is applied to tonify Yin, adjust collaterals and improve vision. The liver and gallbladder acupoints in 4th region, kidney acupoint in 2nd region and spleen acupoint in 7th region are added for deficiency of liver and kidney Yin; and the heart acupoint in 6th region is added for deficiency of heart Yin.

The Chengqi acupoint lies 2 cm below eye and the needle is perpendicularly inserted until its tip reaching the bone; and the Qiuhou acupoint lies at the junction of lateral one fourth and medial 3 fourths of lower orbital border and the needle is slowly inserted into the orbit and immediately removed without twisting, lifting and thrusting stimulation and retention of needle.

(4) Clinical experience

The acupuncture with an adequate technique and a long therapeutic course may produce certain effect, if combined with other therapies. For protecting the eyeball while inserting needle at Chengqi and Qiuhou acupoints, it should be gently pushed upward.

50. Tinnitus and deafness

The tinnitus is a subjective symptom with a ringing noise in ear, the slight deafness is called Zhongting (hard of hearing) with reduction of hearing power to some extent and the severe patients of deafness may completely lose their hearing power. The tinnitus is often a predromal symptom of deafness and they usually occur together.

(1) Etiology and pathogenesis

The tinnitus and deafness are caused by mental depression, poor dispersion of liver qi, transformation of stagnated qi to fire and then to wind pathogen; by damage of liver by fury, transformation of excessive Yang to wind pathogen and upward rushing of wind and fire pathogen to attack the ear; by preference for alcohol andgreasy food, accumulation of damp-heat pathogen to produce phlegm, transformation of accumulated phlegm to fire pathogen and adverse ascent of phlegm and fire to block orifices of sense organs; by exhaustion of kidney essence and emptiness of marrow reservoir (brain) due to sexual intemperance or in weak people and chronic patients; or by deficiency and dysfunction of spleen without enough materials to produce qi and blood, emptiness of meridians and blood vessels and poor supply of clear Yang upward to ears.

(2) Differential diagnosis

1) Upward attack of liver and gallbladder fire: The patients may suffer from sudden onset of tinnitus and deafness, headache, vertigo, flushing face, bitter

taste in mouth, dryness in throat, annoyance, exacerbation of tinnitus and deafness by anger, red tongue proper with yellow coating and stringy rapid pulse.

2) Accumulation of phlegm and fire pathogen: The patients may suffer from tinnitus as chirping of cicada, blocking sensation in ear, chest distress, profuse sputum, bitter taste in mouth, yellow, thin and greasy tongue coating and stringy slippery pulse.

3) Deficiency of kidney essence: The patients may suffer from tinnitus and deafness for a long time, dizziness, vertigo, soreness of waist, emission of semen, red tongue proper and therady or weak thready pulse.

4) Weakness of spleen and stomach: The patients may suffer from tinnitus and deafness worsened by tiredness, poor appetite, mental tiredness, shortness of breath, white thin tongue coating and thready pulse.

(3) Treatment

The eye acupuncture is applied at liver acupoint in 4th region and upper energizer aucpoint in 3rd region to clear liver fire and remove blockage of orifices of sense organs for upward attack of liver and gallbladder fire type; the acupuncture at stomach and spleen acupoints in 7th region and upper energizer acupoint is applied to clear fire and resolve phlegm for accumulation of phlegm and fire pathogen type; the acupuncture at kidney acupoint in 2nd region and upper energizer acupoint to tonify kidney essence and suppress Yang for deficiency of kidney essence type; and the acupuncture at spleen and stomach acupoints and middle energizer acupoint to tonify spleen qi and upward raise clear Yang for weakness of spleen and stomach type.

The reinforcing technique is' applied for deficient syndrome; and the reducing technique is used for excessive type and the needles are retained for 15 min, once a day for 10 times as a therapeutic course with a rest of 3-5 days between 2 courses.

(4) Clinical experience

The eye acupuncture can produce certain effect to treat the tinnitus and acquired deafness by improving the microcirculation of cochlea and the nutrition of hairy cells, but it is not effective to treat the complete deafness or damage, inward depression, turbidity and thickening of ear drum and the patients should visit the doctors in ENT department for treatment. The speech training is useful for the children of congenital deafness before 3 years of age.

51. Biyuan (sinusitis)

This is a disease of nose with increase of thin or thick nasal excretion discharged by drops and intermittent nasal obstruction. The acute and chronic sinusitis in western medicine can be treated by the following methods.

(1) Etiology and pathogenesis

The Biyuan is caused by invasion of wind-heat pathogen or transformation of wind-cold pathogen into heat pathogen to attack lungs and disturb the clearing and dispersing function of lungs and the upward steaming of heat pathogen in lung to scorch the sinuses of nose; by upward invasion of excessive fire pathogen of liver and gallbladder to attack orifices of sense organs; or by invasion and accumulation of cold pathogen in lungs to block the nose in patients with reduction of lung qi.

(2) Differential diagnosis

1) Wind-cold type: The patients at early stage of acute sinusitis or during acute attack of chronic sinusitis may suffer from chillness, fever, no sweating,

headache, nasal obstruction, discharge of white, clear and thin nasal excretion and white thin tongue coating. After the transformation of cold pathogen to heat pathogen in lungs the patients may suffer from slight mental dullness, high fever, sweating, thirst, pain and distension of head, nasal obstruction, poor smelling sensation, hot breathing air, discharge of profuse yellow sticky nasal excretion, red tongue proper with light yellow coating.

2) Heat pathogen in gallbladder type: The patients may suffer from discharge of yellow or yellowish green, turbid, sticky and foul nasal excretion as pus, poor smelling sensation, headache, annoyance, anger, dizziness, tinnitus, bitter taste in mouth, pain in flanks, red tongue proper with yellow coating.

3) Deficiency of lung qi type: The chronic patients may suffer from discharge of profuse white nasal excretion without bad smell and in a varied thickness, intermittent nasal obstruction, relief of nasal discharge and obstruction by hotness and physical exercise and aggravation of nasal symptoms by stimulation of wind and coldness, weakness of body, shortness of breath, cold body and limbs and pale tongue proper with white slippery coating.

(3) Treatment

To disperse lung qi and release nasal obstruction.

The eye acupuncture is applied at upper energizer acupoint in 3rd region, lung acupoint in 1st region and other acupoints selected according to inspection of blood vessels on eye and the body acupuncture is applied at Yingxiang (LI 20) and Tongtian (BL 7) acupoints.

The reducing or even reinforcing and reducing technique is applied to the patients caused by attack of external pathogens or heat pathogen in gallbladder; and the reinforcing technique is used for the deficiency of lung qi type. Yhe needle is inserted toward the root of nose as the acupuncture applied at Yingxiang acupoint; and the needle is inserted forward at Tongtian acupoint.

(4) Clinical experience

The eye acupuncture can produce an apparent effect on acute sinusitis, but it can only improve some symptoms in chronic sinusitis.

52. Sore throat

The sore throat is a common disease of throat and it is called Houbi (Bi-syndrome of throat) in traditional

Chinese medicine.

(1) Etiology and pathogenesis

The sore throat is caused by invasion of external wind-heat pathogen to scorch the trachea and lungs; by overeating of too much spicy and fried food, upward ascent of stomach fire to produce phlegm by steaming the body fluid and accumulation of phlegm and fire pathogen in throat; or by poor supply of body fluid and upward flaming of deficient fire to scorch throat.

(2) Differential diagnosis

1) Wind-heat type: The onset is prompt and the patients may suffer from redness, swelling and pain in throat, chillness, fever, cough with hoarse voice, blocking sensation in throat, difficulty to swallow, thin tongue coating and floating rapid pulse.

2) Excessive heat type: The patients may suffer from swelling and severe pain in throat, high fever, headache, thirst with desire to drink much water, foul smell from mouth, spitting of yellow sticky sputum, constipation, discharge of dark urine in short stream, yellow thick tongue coating and full rapid pulse.

3) Deficient heat type: The patients may suffer from slight swelling and redness in throat with dull pain or swallowing pain, dryness of tongue and mouth cavi-

ty, red cheeks, tidal fever, hotness in palms and soles, red tongue proper and thready rapid pulse.

(3) Treatment

The lung acupoint in 1st region and upper energizer acupoint in 3rd region are used for sore throat of all types. The eye acupuncture is applied at lung and large intestine acupoints in 1st region and upper energizer acupoint to disperse wind, clear heat and relieve sore throat for wind-heat type; the acupuncture is applied at large intestine acupoint and stomach acupoint in 7th region to clear heat, resolve phlegm and relieve sore throat for excessive heat type; and the acupuncture is applied at kidney acupoint in 2nd region and lung acupoint to tonify Yin, extinguish fire and relieve sore throat for deficient fire type.

The reducing technique is used for the wind-heat and excessive heat types; and the even reinforcing and reducing technique is used for the deficient type. The bleeding therapy may be applied at Shixuan (EX-UE 11) acupoints.

(4) Clinical experience

The eye acupuncture can produce an apparent effect on both acute and chronic sore throat, but the effect is better in acute sore throat and the chronic sore throat needs a longer therapeutic course. The bleeding therapy can improve the therapeutic result of eye acupuncture. The patients should be further examined to rule out any serious diseases if the acupuncture can not produce any effect after a long course of treatment.

53. Toothache

The toothache is a common symptom with the pain induced or exacerbated by the stimulation of coldness, hotness or sour and sweet food and it can be divided into deficient and excessive types. The excessive type is caused by the stomach fire or wind-fire pathogens; and the deficient type is caused by the deficient fire.

(1) Etiology and pathogenesis

The toothache may be caused by invasion of wind pathogen into Yángming meridians and the accumulated wind pathogen can be transformed into fire pathogen to flame up along Yangming meridians to produce wind-fire toothache; by accumulation of stomach fire to upward attack the teeth; or by deficiency of kidney Yin and flaming up of deficient fire to cause toothache.

(2) Differential diagnosis

1) Wind-fire type: The onset of toothache is

prompt with swelling of gum and the patients also suffer from low fever, chillness, white thin tongue coating and floating rapid pulse.

2) Stomach fire type: The patients may suffer from severe toothache, foul smell from mouth, constipation, yellow tongue coating and full stringy pulse.

3) Deficient fire type: The patients may suffer from intermittent dull toothache, loose teeth, dryness in mouth and throat, mental tiredness, soreness of waist, red tongue tip and thready rapid pulse.

(3) Treatment

The upper energizer acupoint in 3rd region is used to do eye acupuncture, and Yifeng (TE 17, in a depression behind earlobe) acupoint on the diseased side is used to do body acupuncture.

The eye acupuncture is applied at large intestine acupoint in 1st region and middle energizer acupoint in 5th region to expel wind pathogen, clear heat pathogen, release blockage of meridians and stop pain for toothache of wind-heat type; the acupuncture is applied at stomach acupoint in 7th region and middle energizer acupoint to clear stomach fire for stomach fire type; and the acupuncture is applied at kidney acupoint in 2nd region and liver acupoint in 4th region to tonify kidney, subdue hyperactivity of liver and extinguish fire pathogen for deficient fire type.

The reducing technique is applied for excessive toothache; and the reinforcing or even reinforcing and reducing technique is applied for deficient toothache and the needles are retained for 20 min, 1-2 times a day.

(4) Clinical experience

The eye acupuncture can produce a quick effect to stop acute severe toothache, which is often refractory to analgesic administered by mouth. The acupuncture may be used as a supplemental therapy to the dental treatment for caries of tooth with infection, necrotic pulpitis or impacted wisdom tooth. The patients should always keep their oral cavity clean.

54. Febrile diseases

The fever as a common symptom with elevated body temperature may occur in many diseases, including infectious diseases, infection, tumor, allergy and endocrinal disturbance and it can be divided into low and high fever. In this chapter only the fever of infection and infectious diseases is discussed.

(1) Etiology and pathogenesis

The febrile diseases are caused by invasion of wind-cold or wind-heat pathogen through mouth and nose or skin and hair to attack lungs and impair the body resistance and dispersing function of lungor by invasion of epidemic or toxic-heat pathogen into qi or blood and even directly into Yangming meridians to produce epilepsy and convulsion.

(2) Differential diagnosis

1) Attack of pathogen to Wei (defensive energy): The patients may suffer from fever, chillness, no sweating, headache, pain in body, nasal obstruction, cough, sore throat, white thin tongue coating and floating rapid pulse.

2) Attack of pathogen to qi: The patients may suffer from high fever, no chillness, sweating, thirst, cough, spitting of yellow sticky sputum, discharge of dark urine, flushing face, yellow greasy tongue coating and full rapid pulse.

3) Attack of pathogen to Ying (nutritive material): The patients may suffer from high fever, thirst without desire to drink much water, restlessness, mental confusion, red tongue proper with yellow greasy coating and thready rapid pulse.

4) Attack of pathogen to blood: The patients may

suffer from high fever, restlessness, coma, delirium, convulsion of limbs and even hemoptysis and nasal bleeding, dark crimson tongue proper and thready rapid pulse.

(3) Treatment

The eye acupuncture is applied at lung and large intestine acupoints in 1st region to expel pathogen from body surface and disperse lung qi for febrile diseases of pathogen in Wei type; the acupuncture is applied at large intestine acupoint in 1st region and stomach acupoint in 7th region to clear heat pathogen for pathogen in qi type; the body accupuncture is applied at Shixuan (EX-HN 11) acupoints and 12 Jing (well) acupoints to clear heat and release blockage of orifices of sense organs for pathogen in Ying type; and the eye acupuncture is applied at large intestine acupoint in 1st region, urinary bladder acupoint in 2nd region and spleen acupoint in 7th region to clear heat pathogen in blood for pathogen in blood type.

The reducing technique is applied for patients of all types of febrile diseases and the acupuncture can be applied 1-3 times a day according to the height of body temperature. The bleeding therapy is applied at Shixuan (tops of 10 fingers) and 12 Jing acupoints (the lateral and medial corners of nail of little finger, lateral corner of nail of index finger, medial corner of nail of ring finger and tip of middle finger).

(4) Clinical experience

The eye acupuncture can expel pathogen on body surface and clear heat to treat febrile diseases of pathogen in Wei and qi types; but it can only temporally control the fever and relieve the symptoms of febrile diseases of pathogen in Ying and blood types, which should be treated by their specific effective therapies with acupuncture as a supplemental treatment.

55. Jue-syndrome (syncope)

This is a critical disease with sudden falling down and loss of consciousness. The patients of mild type may have pale complexion and cold limbs; and the severe patients may suffer from mental confusion, loss of consciousness and incontinence of urine and stool.

(1) Etiology and pathogenesis

The syncope may be caused by injury of liver due to mental depression and accumulation of liver qi in heart and chest to interfere the mental activity; by disturbance of circulation of qi due to emotional upset to produce Jue-syndrome of qi type; by upward ascent of liver Yang with qi and blood induced by fury in people with deficiency of kidney Yin and excessiveness of liver Yang to interfere mental activity and produce Jue-syndrome of blood type; by poor supply of Yang qi to brain due to overfatigue in weak people; or by deficiency of qi and blood and emptiness of brain due to loss of much blood to produce sudden syncope.

(2) Differential diagnosis

1) Jue-symptom of qi type: The patients may suddenly fall in syncope induced by mental depression or emotional stimulation, slight mental confusion, presence of sensation, holding breath or rough breath, locked jaw, no word to speak, clenched fist with thumb embraced by other fingers, chest distress, white thin tongue coating and stringy pulse.

2) Jue-syndrome of blood type: The patients may suddenly fall down, loss of consciousness, flushing face, red eyes, locked jaw and induction of symptoms by fury or overfatigue. They may have history of headache, vertigo and hypertension. The tongue proper is redder than normal with yellow thin coating and the pulse is stringy and slippery.

3) Jue-syndrome of syncope type: The patients

may suffer from syncope following the sudden appearance of dizziness, chest distress and nausea and they also have pale complexion, cold limbs, cold sweating, white thin tongue coating and thready pulse.

(3) Treatment

The eye acupuncture is applied at upper energizer acupoint in 3rd region and liver acupoint in 4th region to disperse liver qi for Jue-syndrome of qi type; the acupuncture is applied at liver acupoint and kidney acupoint in 2nd region to induce resuscitation of mind for Jue-syndrome of blood type; and the acupuncture is applied at upper energizer acupoint in 3rd region and lower energizer acupoint in 8th region to recover Yang qi and rescue collapse for Jue-syndrome of syncope type.

The reducing technique is applied for Jue-syndrome of qi or blood type; and the reinforcing technique is applied for Jue-syndrome of syncope type. The moxibustion with moxa cones is applied at Qihai (CV 6), Guanyuan (CV 4) and Shenque (CV 8) acupoints and the moxibustion with moxa roll is applied at Baihui (GV 20) acupoint.

(4) Clinical experience

The strong stimulation of acupuncture is applied to patients of Jue-syndrome of qi type for resuscitation of mind; a combined therapy should be used to treat Jue-syndrome of blood type; and the finger-pressing method is used to treat the mild syncope. The patients should keep a calm mood and stable emotion.

56. Jing-syndrome (epilepsy)

The Jing-syndrome is a severe disease with convulsion of limbs, stiffness of neck and back, opisthotonos, upward staring of eyes and coma.

(1) Etiology and pathogenesis

The Jing-syndrome is caused by stirring up of liver wind due to attack of violent heat pathogen, deficiency of blood or formation of endogenous wind from excessive Yang.

(2) Differential diagnosis

1) Excessiveness of Yang type: The patients may suffer from headache, dizziness, numbness of limbs, slurred speech, convulsion of limbs, sudden falling down, unconsciousness, red tongue proper with white thin coating and stringy pulse.

2) Violent heat pathogen type: The patients may suffer from persistent high fever, thirst with desire to drink water, red face and eyes, convulsion of limbs,

upward staring of eyes, coma, stiffness of neck and back, red tongue proper with yellow coating and full rapid pulse.

3) Deficiency of blood type: The patients may suffer from headache, dizziness, mental clearness, tremor or slight convulsion of limbs, pale tongue proper with white thin coating and thready pulse.

(3) Treatment

The even reinforcing and reducing technique of eye acupuncture is applied at liver acupoint in 4th region and kidney acupoint in 2nd region to subdue hyperactive liver and calm down wind for excessive Yang type; the reducing technique is applied at large intestine acupoint in 1st region and spleen acupoint in 7th region to clear heat and calm down wind for violent heat type; and the reinforcing technique is applied at heart acupoint in 6th region, liver and spleen acupoints to nourish liver and calm down wind for blood deficiency type. The acupuncture is applied 1-2 time a day for the former 2 types and once a day for the last type.

(4) Clinical experience

The acupuncture can produce an apparent effect to control convulsion, but it may relapse if the etiological factors have not been eliminated.

57. Tong-syndrome (painful diseases)

The pain in body with varied intensity may be cuased by invasion of external pathogens or emotional disturbance to block the circulation of qi and blood. In this chapter only the severe pain in triple energizer regions is discussed.

(1) Etiology and pathogenesis

The upper energizer contains heart and lungs and the pain in upper energizer is due to reduction of Yang and accumulation of phlegm in chest caused by invasion of cold pathogen and dysfunction of spleen; the middle energizer contains liver, gallbladder, spleen and stomach and the pain in middle energizer is due to deficiency of spleen and stomach Yang and blockage of circulation of qi caused by improper diet and emotional disturbance; and the lower energizer contains kidney, urinary bladder, uterus and intestine and the pain in lower energizer is due to stagnation of qi and blood caused by invasion of cold and summer damp-heat pathogens, overeating of food or emotional disturbance.

(2) Differential diagnosis

1) Pain in upper energizer: The patients may suf-

fer from fixed pain in heart and chest radiated to left shoulder and arm, sweating, cold limbs, pale complexion, purple lips and tongue proper with white thin coating and stringy thready pulse.

2) Pain in middle energizer: The patients may suffer from persistent pain in upper abdomen, annoyance, anger, dryness and bitter taste in mouth, white or yellow, thin and greasy tongue coating and stringy pulse.

3) Pain in lower energizer: The patients may suffer from severe colic pain in lower abdomen to cause repeated turning over of body in bed, cold hands and feet, cold sweating, preference for hotness and pressure applied to lower abdomen, white thin tongue coating and stringy tense pulse.

(3) Treatment

The eye acupuncture is applied at upper energizer acupoint in 3rd region and lung acupoint in 1st region to expand chest, adjust circulation of qi, release blood stasis and relieve pain for pain in upper energizer; the acupuncture is applied at middle energizer aucpoint in 5th region, spleen acupoint in 7th region and liver and gallbladder acupoints in 4th region to disperse liver qi, relieve spasm and stop pain for pain in middle energizer; and the acupuncture is applied at lower energizer acupoint in 8th region, spleen acupoint in 7th region and liver acupoint in 4th region to warm internal organs, expel cold pathogen and release stagnation of liver qi for pain in lower energizer. The painful diseases are all of the excessive syndrome, the reducing technique is therefore used for all of them.

(4) Clinical experience

The eye acupuncture can relieve the acute pain caused by spasm of stomach, renal colic, dysmenorrhea and biliary colic.

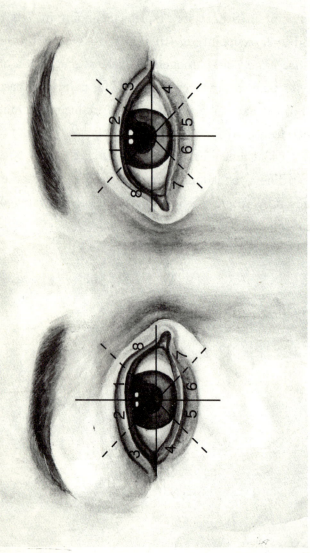

图书在版编目(CIP)数据

眼针疗法：英文/赵昕主编；王台翻译．
－北京：学苑出版社，1997.8
ISBN 7-5077-1364-4
Ⅰ．眼… Ⅱ．①赵… ②王… Ⅲ．眼针疗法 Ⅳ．R77
中国版本图书馆CIP数据核字（97）第18014号

眼针疗法

赵昕主编

王台翻译

学苑出版社
（中国北京万寿路西街11号）
邮政编码 100036
北京大兴沙窝店印刷厂印刷
中国国际图书贸易总公司发行
（中国北京车公庄西路35号）
北京邮政信箱第399号 邮政编码100044
英文版 32 开本
ISBN 7-5077-1364-4

04000
14-E-3137P